MRCPsych Pap

600 MCQs

MRCPsych Paper 1

600 MCQs

Ashok G Patel MBBS DPM FRCPsych
Consultant General Adult Psychiatrist (Retired)
South Essex Partnership University NHS Foundation Trust
Luton, UK

Roshelle Ramkisson MBBS MRCPsych MSc (Health and Public
Leadership) PGDip Psychiatry MDCH
Consultant Psychiatrist in Child and Adolescent Psychiatry
Pennine Care NHS Foundation Trust
Royal Oldham Hospital
Oldham, UK

Raman Sharma MBBS MSc (Psychiatric Practice) MRCPsych
Specialty Doctor in Psychiatry
South Essex Partnership University NHS Foundation Trust
Bedford Hospital
Bedford, UK

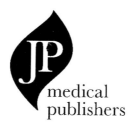

JP
medical
publishers

London • Philadelphia • Panama City • New Delhi

© 2014 JP Medical Ltd.
Published by JP Medical Ltd,
83 Victoria Street, London, SW1H 0HW, UK
Tel: +44 (0)20 3170 8910
Fax: +44 (0)20 3008 6180
Email: info@jpmedpub.com
Web: www.jpmedpub.com

ISBN: 978-1-907816-39-0

British Library Cataloguing in Publication Data
A catalogue record for this book is available from the British Library

Library of Congress Cataloging in Publication Data
A catalog record for this book is available from the Library of Congress

JP Medical Ltd is a subsidiary of Jaypee Brothers Medical Publishers (P) Ltd, New Delhi, India

Commissioning Editor: Steffan Clements
Design: Designers Collective Ltd

Typeset, printed and bound in India.

Preface

The MRCPsych examinations are extremely challenging, and candidates must be meticulous in their preparation if they are to stand any chance of success. Understanding this principle has been fundamental during our preparation of this book, and we have endeavoured to provide sufficient MCQ revision material for each element of the curriculum. We are confident that by using this book, readers will be well armed to face the MCQ component of the Paper 1 exam.

In order to facilitate revision, we have mapped the questions in the first four chapters to the curriculum topics. The fifth chapter is intentionally unstructured, and has been included to provide a mock exam representative of the MCQ component of Paper 1, which readers can use to practise under exam conditions. All questions are based on the curriculum and thorough answers have been provided to explain the rationale behind each correct answer option.

The burden of editorship has been wisely spread to harness varied expertise. In psychiatry, innovation in practice tends to be evolutionary rather than revolutionary, and much of our knowledge remains to be translated into practical innovations in patient care. It is our intention that this book will help psychiatry trainees not only to pass the MRCPsych Paper 1 examination, but also to improve their patient care. We believe that the book will assist trainees, trainers, educational and clinical supervisors, College tutors, Directors of Medical Education, SAS tutors and Training Programme Directors in preparation for the MRCPsych examinations.

Ashok G Patel
Roshelle Ramkisson
Raman Sharma
December 2013

Contents

Acknowledgements

We would like to thank the colleagues and friends who have helped us as we prepared this book. They have been a great source of useful advice and suggestions and have read the draft papers to make sure that the questions and answers were compatible with the MRCPsych Paper 1 exam.

We are also most grateful to the many people behind the scenes without whose help this book would not have been possible. In particular, we would like to thank the publishers, especially Steffan Clements, Hannah Applin and Katrina Rimmer for their encouragement and support from the very beginning to the end of the project. Special thanks go to Sue Keely and Mrs Vasanthi Varadharajan in preparing the manuscripts.

We would like to thank Nicola Cowdery, Deepak Garg, Vineel Reddy, Khurram Sadiq, Ajaya Upadhyaya, Dinesh Khanna, Faisal Pervez, Sanjith Kamath, Vishelle Kamath, Basavaraja Papanna and Juhi Mishra for their support and encouragement.

Finally, we would also like to thank the families of the authors and our own families for putting up with us as inevitably the book has been written during evenings, weekends and holidays.

AP, RR, RS

Lead Contributing Authors

Gursharan Lal Kashyap MBBS DCH MD MRCPsych
Chapter 2: Questions and Answers
Specialist Registrar Year 5 in Psychiatry
South Essex Partnership University NHS
Foundation Trust
Bedford Hospital
Bedford, UK

Jon van Niekerk MBChB MRCPsych
Chapter 3: Questions and Answers
Consultant Psychiatrist
Greater Manchester West Mental Health NHS
Foundation Trust
Royal Bolton Hospital
Bolton, UK

Komal A Patel BSc MBChB MRCS
Chapter 1: Questions and Answers
Core Trainee Year 2 in Surgery
Surrey & Sussex Healthcare NHS Trust
East Surrey Hospital
Redhill, UK

Vineel Reddy MBBS MRCPsych
Chapter 4: Questions and Answers
Speciality Trainee Year 5 in Liaison Psychiatry
Countess of Chester Hospital NHS Foundation
Trust
Chester, UK

Madhavan Seshadri MBBS DPM MRCPsych
Chapter 5: Questions
Specialist Registrar Year 6 in Psychiatry
South Essex Partnership University NHS
Foundation Trust
Bedford, UK

Samir Shah MBBS MRCPsych MSc
Chapter 3: Questions and Answers
Consultant Psychiatrist in General Adult
Psychiatry
Cheshire and Wirral Partnership NHS
Foundation Trust
Macclesfield, UK

Raman Sharma MBBS MSc (Psychiatric
Practice) MRCPsych
Chapter 1: Questions and Answers
Specialty Doctor in Psychiatry
South Essex Partnership University NHS
Foundation Trust
Bedford Hospital
Bedford, UK

Kishan Sharma MBBS MRCPsych
Chapter 4: Questions and Answers
Consultant Child and Adolescent Psychiatrist
Trafford Healthcare NHS Trust
Manchester, UK

Ankush Singhal MBBS MD MRCPsych
Chapter 2: Questions and Answers
Consultant Liaison Psychiatrist
Pennine Care NHS Foundation Trust
The Royal Oldham Hospital
Oldham, UK

Baljit Kaur Upadhyay MBBS
Chapter 5: Questions and Answers
Specialty Doctor in Psychiatry
South Essex Partnership University NHS
Foundation Trust
Luton, UK

Contributors

Syed Ashraf MBBS PGCHM
Specialty Doctor in Psychiatry
South Essex Partnership University NHS
Foundation Trust
Bedford Hospital
Bedford, UK

Nicola Cowdery MBChB MRCPsych MSc
Specialty Trainee Year 5 in General Adult Psy-
chiatry
Greater Manchester West Mental Health NHS
Foundation Trust
Prestwich Hospital
Manchester, UK

Chapter 1

Test questions: 1

Questions: MCQs

For each question, select one answer option.

HISTORY AND MENTAL STATE EXAMINATION

1. A 69-year-old woman presented with severe depression and short-term memory problems. Which of the following tests is most appropriate to assess her short-term memory?

   A Copying a clock
   B Copying pentagons
   C Orientation to time and place
   D Serial sevens
   E Three-word recall

2. Which of the following statements regarding frontal lobe dysfunction is correct?

   A The ability to plan ahead is preserved
   B Agnosia is a diagnostic feature
   C Dyscalculia is often present
   D Long-term memory loss is a consistent feature
   E Perseveration is a sign of a frontal lobe lesion

3. A 70-year-old man undertakes a Mini-Mental State Examination (MMSE). He asks what is being assessed when he is instructed to take away serial 7s from 100 and then repeat the result. Which of the following is the most appropriate response?

   A Attention
   B Language
   C Remote memory
   D Verbal memory
   E Working memory

4. Which of the following statements regarding epileptic automatism is correct?

   A Consciousness is preserved
   B The control of posture is lost
   C An epileptic automatism lasts from seconds to minutes
   D The muscle tone is preserved
   E The recall of events is accurate

5. Which of the following about Ganser's syndrome is correct?

   A Accurate answers
   B Amnesia of the episode

C   Clear consciousness
D   Orientation to time and person
E   Right–left disorientation

6. A 21-year-old man takes a large number of paracetamol tablets with alcohol after an argument with his girlfriend. On examination, he displays fluctuating consciousness, irritable mood, agitation, restlessness and impaired concentration. His MMSE score is 22/30. What is the most likely diagnosis?

A   Acute psychotic episode
B   Acute stress reaction
C   Adjustment disorder
D   Delirium
E   Panic disorder

COGNITIVE ASSESSMENT

7. A 62-year-old man presents with significant cognitive impairment accompanied by disinhibition, recklessness and a lack of concern towards others. Taking into consideration the type of dementia that he might have, which of the following language deficits could this patient experience initially?

A   Dysarthria
B   Dyslexia
C   Fluent expressive dysphasia
D   Non-fluent expressive dysphasia
E   Receptive dysphasia

8. Which of the following conditions is commonly associated with a catastrophic reaction?

A   Bipolar affective disorder
B   Borderline personality disorder
C   Cocaine misuse
D   Schizophrenia
E   Vascular dementia

9. Which of the following is a test for working memory?

A   The behavioural inattention test
B   The Hayling and Brixton tests
C   The token test
D   The trail making test
E   The zoo map

10. Which of the following is a non-verbal performance component of the Wechsler adult intelligence scale (WAIS)?

A   Arithmetic
B   Comprehension
C   Digit span
D   Matrix reasoning
E   Similarities

11. A 70-year-old woman was assessed in the memory assessment clinic. She was asked about the Royal wedding in 2011, which she found difficult to answer. Which part of her memory was being tested?

A   Immediate
B   Procedural

C   Recent
D   Remote
E   Working

12. A 32-year-old man was seen following a road traffic accident. He was confused, but he opened his eyes on painful stimuli. On the Glasgow coma score (GCS) scale, what is his eye-opening grade?

A   1
B   2
C   3
D   4
E   5

13. Which of the following tests measures intelligence that is relatively independent of educational background?

A   The California verbal learning test
B   The Cambridge contextual reading test
C   The national adult reading test
D   Raven's progressive matrices
E   The Wechsler abbreviated scale of intelligence

14. In which of the following conditions are the NINDS-AIREN criteria useful in their diagnosis?

A   Alzheimer's dementia
B   Dementia due to normal pressure hydrocephalus
C   Lewy body dementia
D   Parkinson's dementia complex
E   Vascular dementia

15. Which of the following is a verbal component of the WAIS?

A   Arithmetic
B   Block design
C   Digit symbol
D   Matrix reasoning
E   Picture completion

NEUROLOGICAL EXAMINATION

16. A 45-year-old man undergoes a routine physical examination. He previously had retrobulbar neuritis in his left eye, from which he apparently made complete recovery. What is the most likely sign on examination of the pupils?

A   An irregular left pupil
B   Left pupil completely unreactive to light
C   Unilateral pupillary constriction on the left with slight ptosis
D   When light shone back to the left eye from the right, the pupil dilates
E   When light shone in the right eye both pupils dilate

17. A 25-year-old man presented with impairment of auditory comprehension and repetition. He had an intact speech and an intact ability to write and read. Which of the following is the most likely presenting feature?

A   Broca's aphasia
B   Pure agraphia

    C   Pure word blindness
    D   Pure word deafness
    E   Wernicke's aphasia

18. A 61-year-old man developed bitemporal hemianopia. Where is the lesion most likely to be located?

    A   Left optic tract
    B   Optic chiasma
    C   Occipital lobe
    D   Right optic nerve
    E   Right optic radiation

19. A 29-year-old African man presented to the emergency department confused and irritable, with a headache and a high temperature. He is HIV positive and MRI of the brain showed multiple ring-shaped lesions. What is the most likely diagnosis?

    A   Cryptococal meningitis
    B   Cytomegalovirus encephalitis
    C   Progressive multifocal leukoencephalopathy
    D   Toxoplasma encephalitis
    E   Viral meningitis

ASSESSMENT

20. A 39-year-old woman presented with depression, apathy, weakness, fatigue and loss of weight. On clinical examination, she had areas of pigmentation on her body. A blood test revealed hypokalaemia. Which of the following is most likely to be found on further investigation?

    A   Abnormal Synacthen test
    B   Acanthosis
    C   Hyponatraemia
    D   Low serum ceruloplasmin
    E   Low vitamin B_6

21. A 19-year-old woman presents with emotional lability, behavioural disturbance and stiffness of joints. On examination she has mild jaundice and hepatomegaly. An MRI of the brain showed cortical atrophy and hypodense areas in the basal ganglia. Which of the following will be seen on further investigation?

    A   Decreased 24-hour urinary copper
    B   Decreased hepatic copper
    C   Increased total serum copper
    D   Increased free serum copper
    E   Increased serum ceruloplasmin

22. A 44-year-old woman presented with severe panic attacks, pronounced tachycardia, headache and vomiting. In between these episodes, she reported feeling exhausted. On clinical examination, her blood pressure was 175/105. On investigation, her blood glucose was elevated. Which of the following is most likely to be found on further investigation?

    A   Hypokalaemia
    B   Hyponatraemia
    C   Low folic acid
    D   Low vitamin B_{12}
    E   Raised urinary catecholamine

23. You are asked to assess an 80-year-old widow in primary care whose family tells you that they cannot manage her at home, as she has been verbally abusive and threatening. Which of the following neuropsychological tests would be most appropriate to assess her mood?

    A   General health questionnaire
    B   Geriatric depression scale
    C   Mini-mental state examination
    D   Present state examination
    E   Wisconsin card sorting test

24. You are asked to assess an 80-year-old widow whose family tells you that they cannot manage her at home, as she has been verbally abusive and threatening. Which of the following neuropsychological tests is most appropriate to assess if the patient had a global deterioration in her cognition?

    A   Burden interview
    B   Clinical dementia rating scale
    C   Clock-drawing test
    D   Hachinski's ischaemia score
    E   Mini-mental state examination

25. You are asked to assess an 80-year-old widow whose family tells you that they cannot manage her at home as she has been aggressive and threatening towards them. Her global cognition is within normal range. Which of the following tests would be most appropriate to assess whether she had a specific frontal lobe deficit?

    A   Clinical dementia rating scale
    B   Hachinski's ishaemia score
    C   Mini-mental state examination
    D   Quality of life – Alzheimer's disease scale
    E   Wisconsin card sorting test

26. A 50-year-old divorced man was rushed to the emergency department when he was found to be confused and vomiting at home. He has a long history of alcohol abuse and presented with a patchy history about his problems. He complained of severe difficulties with his vision and walking. A diagnosis of Wernicke's encephalopathy is considered. Which of the following features would help to confirm the diagnosis?

    A   Acalculia
    B   Apathy
    C   Finger agnosia
    D   Ophthalmoplegia
    E   Peripheral neuropathy

27. A 59-year-old man with a long history of alcohol abuse was referred to the outpatient clinic for psychiatric assessment. He complained of memory problems with periods of mental confusion for several months. A diagnosis of Korsakoff's syndrome is considered. Which of the following features will help to confirm the diagnosis?

    A   Acalculia
    B   Anterograde amnesia
    C   Aphasia
    D   Euphoria
    E   Retrograde amnesia

28. A 25-year-old single man presented to the outpatient clinic. He suddenly became very threatening and potentially violent towards the doctor. What is the most appropriate action to manage the immediate situation?

    A   Attempt to restrain the patient
    B   Calmly leave the interview room

C   Confront the patient about his behaviour
D   Ensure that you collect all the necessary clinical information before leaving
E   Ignore the patient's behaviour and continue assessing him

29. A 35-year-old, recently separated man presented to the emergency department having taken an overdose of 45 paracetamol tablets. What is the single most significant factor used to assess his current suicide risk?

A   Employment status
B   Gender
C   Marital status
D   Mental status
E   Overdose when alone in hotel room

AETIOLOGY

30. Some individuals are genetically predisposed to particular complications of alcohol misuse. Which enzyme deficiency is implicated in development of organic brain complications?

A   Alcohol dehydrogenase
B   Aldehyde dehydrogenase
C   Guanylyl cyclase
D   Phospholipase A_2
E   Transketolase

31. Which of the following parental styles is the strongest predictor of future offending?

A   Cold emotional relationships
B   Limited parental involvement
C   Limited parental reinforcement
D   Poor discipline
E   Poor parental supervision

32. Which of the following is most likely to be associated with attention deficit hyperactivity disorder in a 14-year-old girl?

A   Behaviourally inhibited temperament
B   Enmeshment in family
C   Functional abnormalities in the prefrontal area
D   Parental divorce
E   Rise in oestrogen levels in female puberty

33. Which pathophysiological factor is most likely related to the reward mechanism in alcohol abuse?

A β-Amyloid precursor protein
B   Mammillary body α-ketoglutarate
C   Subcortical leukomalacia
D   Tau protein
E   Ventral tegmental area dopamine and enkephalin

34. Which of the following is most highly determined by behavioural patterns at 10 years of age?

A   Alcohol misuse
B   Antisocial behaviour
C   Bulimia nervosa
D   Depression
E   Drug abuse

35. Which of the following is most likely to be associated with an increased risk of developing schizophrenia?

    A   Being born in an urban area
    B   Being recurrently placed in a 'double-bind' situation as a child
    C   Experiencing high expressed emotions in the family home
    D   Maternal alcohol use during pregnancy
    E   Maternal cannabis use during pregnancy

DIAGNOSIS

36. An 80-year-old man has developed bilateral cataracts over the past few years. He is physically well. However, he presented with increased paranoia over the past 6 months. He has been observed talking to imaginary people in his room. What is the most likely diagnosis?

    A   Charles Bonnet syndrome
    B   Delirium tremens
    C   Dementia
    D   Diogenes syndrome
    E   Frégoli syndrome

37. A 30-year-old single woman developed rapid onset of bad dreams and nightmares with increased startle reaction. She has difficulty in relaxing and sustaining attention. Her symptoms are worse at night. What is the most likely diagnosis?

    A   Acute stress reaction
    B   Delirium
    C   Generalised anxiety disorder
    D   Post-traumatic stress disorder
    E   Somnambulism

38. A 35-year-old woman has been feeling anxious and distressed following a road traffic accident. She has reduced awareness of her surroundings and experiences symptoms of dissociation. She is fearful and transiently disoriented. What is the most likely diagnosis?

    A   Acute stress reaction
    B   Adjustment disorder
    C   Generalised anxiety disorder
    D   Intracranial bleed
    E   Post-traumatic stress disorder

39. A 50-year-old man experienced a traumatic event while travelling on public transport. He started to experience fragments of images and memories of the event 6 months after the incident. He has sleep disruptions with nightmares and distressing dreams. He avoids going out and gets panicky when he has to use public transport. What is the most likely diagnosis?

    A   Acute stress reaction
    B   Adjustment disorder
    C   Agoraphobia
    D   Dissociative disorder
    E   Post-traumatic stress disorder

CLASSIFICATION

40. According to the *International Classification of Disease*, 10th revision (ICD-10), which category describes neurasthenia?

    A   Adjustment disorders
    B   Dissociative disorders
    C   Other anxiety disorders
    D   Other neurotic disorders
    E   Somatoform disorders

41. Which of the following statements with regard to ICD-10 classification is correct?

    A   Operational classification system
    B   Rigid in its definitions
    C   Suitable for research purposes
    D   More user friendly than the DSM-IV
    E   Widely used in USA

42. Which of the following statements distinguishes the *Diagnostic and Statistical Manual* of *Mental Disorders*, 4th edn (DSM-IV) from the ICD-10?

    A   Bipolar I and bipolar II are differentiated in the ICD-10
    B   Borderline personality disorder is classified as impulsive and borderline in the ICD-10
    C   Personality disorder is classified on a separate axis in the DSM-IV
    D   Recurrent brief depressive disorder is a new addition to the DSM-IV
    E   Schizotypal disorder is with personality disorders in the DSM-IV

43. Which of the following statements regarding the differences between the ICD-10 and the DSM-IV is correct?

    A   The ICD-10 has one version whereas the DSM-IV has different versions
    B   The ICD-10 is available in English only whereas the DSM-IV is available in all widely spoken languages
    C   The ICD-10 is a five-axis system classification whereas the DSM-IV is a three-axis classification
    D   The ICD-10 was developed by the World Health Organization whereas the DSM-IV was developed by the American Psychiatric Association
    E   The ICD-10 includes social consequences of disorders whereas the DSM-IV includes only clinical consequences of disorder

44. Which of the following is included in axis V of the DSM-IV classification?

    A   General medical conditions
    B   Global assessment of functioning
    C   Learning disabilities
    D   Personality disorders
    E   Psychosocial and environmental problems

BASIC PSYCHOPHARMACOLOGY

45. Which of the following statements regarding the pharmacokinetic properties of diazepam is correct?

    A   Desmethyldiazepam is an active metabolite
    B   Its elimination half-life is 10 times greater in elderly people than in young adults

C   The presence of food reduces the extent of its absorption
D   There is 95% protein binding
E   There is 50% bioavailability after oral administration

46. Which of the following statements regarding the physiological effects of benzodiazepines at therapeutic doses is correct?

A   Neuroendocrine systems are affected
B   Stimulation of the afferent pathway results in muscle relaxation
C   The dexamethasone suppression test is unaffected
D   They have little effects on autonomic functions
E   They induce hepatic microsomal enzymes

47. Which of the following statements regarding the pharmacokinetics of psychotropic drugs is correct?

A   First-order kinetics is a non-reversible reaction
B   The concentration of an intravenously administered drug declines exponentially
C   The metabolism of alcohol follows first-order kinetics
D   The term 'bioavailability' refers to the fraction of drug that has been metabolised
E   Two dose forms of the same drug with an equal bioavailability are bioequivalent

48. Which drug should be prescribed with caution in conjunction with fluvoxamine?

A   Amitriptyline
B   Amlodipine
C   Chlorpromazine
D   Naproxen
E   Paracetamol

49. A 30-year-old man was stable on regular antipsychotic medication until 4 days ago when he was admitted with a severe acute psychotic episode. Since then, he has developed hyperpyrexia, muscular rigidity, profuse sweating and disorientation. What is the most likely diagnosis?

A   Akathisia
B   Dystonic reaction
C   Extrapyramidal side effects
D   Neuroleptic malignant syndrome
E   Serotonin syndrome

50. Which of the following is the most common side effect of acamprosate?

A   Hair loss
B   Headache
C   Nausea
D   Stomach cramps
E   Vomiting

51. Which statement regarding serotonin ($5\text{-HT}_2\text{A}$) agonism is correct?

A 5-HT_{2A}-receptors decrease extrapyramidal side effects
B 5-HT_{2A}-receptors have no role in sleep regulation
C 5-HT_{2A}-receptors increase dopamine release
D 5-HT_{2A}-receptors increase glutamate release
E 5-HT_{2A}-receptors inhibit cortical pyramidal neurons

52. Which of the following noradrenergic receptors is presynaptic?

A α_1
B α_2

C α_1
D β_2
E β_3

53. Which of the following statements regarding monoamine interactions in the central nervous system is correct?

A   Noradrenaline can control serotonin release only using feedback inhibition
B   Serotonin has bidirectional control of noradrenaline release
C   Stimulation of 5-HT$_2$A-receptors leads to noradrenaline release
D   Stimulation of α_1-receptors leads to serotonin release
E   Stimulation of α_2-receptors leads to serotonin release

54. What is the most likely mechanism of action of mirtazapine?

A   5-HT$_{2A}$-receptor agonism
B   5-HT$_{2C}$-receptor agonism
C α_2-Receptor agonism
D α_2-Receptor antagonism
E   Blocking serotonin reuptake

55. Which of the following neurotransmitters does venlafaxine act on?

A   Dopamine only
B   Noradrenaline only
C   Serotonin and noradrenaline only
D   Serotonin, noradrenaline and dopamine
E   Serotonin only

56. Which of the following drugs is a dopamine-2 (D_2) antagonist?

A   Amitriptyline
B   Buspirone
C   Diazepam
D   Fluoxetine
E   Zolpidem

57. Which of the following drugs is most useful in the treatment of Gilles de la Tourette's syndrome?

A   Amitriptyline
B   Carbamazepine
C   Dexamphetamine
D   Haloperidol
E   Methylphenidate

BASIC PSYCHOLOGICAL PROCESSES

58. Which of the following is the gestalt determinant of grouping?

A   Delusional set
B   Discontinuation
C   Dissimilarity
D   Figure–ground differentiation
E   Irreversible figures

59. A 5-year-old boy is unable to see the world from his father's point of view and his thinking is dominated by his own perspective. Which stage of Piaget's cognitive development does this best describe?

A   Concrete operational stage
B   Formal operational stage
C   Postconventional stage
D   Preoperational stage
E   Sensorimotor stage

60. A 13-year-old boy has developed logical thinking and the ability to test a hypothesis. At which stage of Piaget's cognitive development is the boy most likely to be?

A   Concrete operational stage
B   Formal operational stage
C   Preconventional stage
D   Preoperational stage
E   Sensorimotor stage

61. An 18-month-old boy discovers that he can make things happen. According to Piaget's cognitive development, which phenomenon of sensorimotor stage has this boy developed?

A   Centation
B   Circular reaction
C   Egocentrism
D   Object permanence
E   Symbolic thought

62. An 8-year-old boy refuses to go out with his friends and says that he will not go out because he does not want to be punished by his parents. At which stage of Kohlberg's model of development is the boy most likely to be?

A   Conventional morality
B   Maintaining social order and law
C   Postconventional morality
D   Preconventional morality
E   Universal principle of justice

63. A 13-year-old boy always does the right thing because he wants people to like him. At which stage of Kohlberg's model of development is the boy most likely to be?

A   Conventional morality
B   Maintaining social order and law
C   Postconventional morality
D   Preconventional morality
E   Universal principle of justice

64. A child starts to say understandable single words, such as 'mummy', 'papa', 'doggie'. What is the most likely age of this child?

A   3 months
B   9 months
C   12 months
D   18 months
E   24 months

65. A girl has recently developed a fear of cats and dogs on the street. She has never behaved like this in the past. What is the most likely age of the girl?

    A   3 years
    B   5 years
    C   5 years plus
    D   10 years age
    E   Teenage onwards

66. A boy used to pick things using his whole palm and all his fingers, but now he picks up objects using his index finger and thumb. What is his most likely age?

    A   2 months
    B   3 months
    C   5 months
    D   6 months
    E   9 months

67. A boy is going through the life stage of initiative versus guilt and has a fear of punishment. According to Erikson's stages of psychosocial development, what is his most likely age group?

    A   0–18 months
    B   18 months to 3 years
    C   3–5 years
    D   6–11 years
    E   12–18 years

HUMAN PSYCHOLOGICAL DEVELOPMENT

68. According to Mary Ainsworth's strange situation procedure, a 15-month-old infant tends not to protest or be distressed when the infant's mother leaves the room, and on reunion he or she ignores her and focuses on the environment. Which of the following best describes this attachment pattern?

    A   Ambivalent
    B   Anxious avoidant
    C   Disorganised
    D   Resistant
    E   Secure

69. Which of the following occurs before the onset of object constancy?

    A   Conventional morality stage
    B   Oral phase
    C   Sensorimotor stage
    D   Separation anxiety
    E   Stranger anxiety

70. Which of the following is most closely associated with the New York longitudinal study by Thomas and Chess?

    A   Attachment
    B   Imprinting
    C   Object constancy
    D   Temperament
    E   Theory of mind

71. Which of the following is included in sensori motor stage of Piaget's cognitive development?

    A   Animistic thinking
    B   Conservation
    C   Egocentric thinking
    D   Object permanence
    E   Transitive inference

72. Which of the following statements about cognitive development is correct?

    A   Each stage is a prerequisite for the next stage of development
    B   Cognitive development is described by Jean Piaget in six stages
    C   It is described by Mary Ainsworth in four stages
    D   It leads to capacity for infant thought processes
    E   It pertains to monkeys as described by Harry Harlow

73. Which of the following statements about learning is correct?

    A   Classic conditioning results from a person's actions
    B   Learning is defined as a change in cognitive functioning
    C   Operant learning is a result of environmental events
    D   Social learning incorporates both classic and operant models
    E   There are several types of learning processes

74. Which of the following statements about learning theory is correct?

    A   Aversive conditioning punishment is used to reduce the frequency of target behaviour
    B   Classic conditioning is the association of a neutral stimulus with a conditioned stimulus, which brings the response originally elicited by an unconditioned stimulus
    C   In habituation, the response to a repeated stimulus increases over time
    D   In operant conditioning, behaviour frequency is altered by observational learning
    E   Instrumental learning means something that is pivotal in the learning process

SOCIAL PSYCHOLOGY

75. A 37-year-old man was overlooked for a job position that he really wanted. He told himself that he did not want the job because of the long hours and burden of responsibility. This is an example of cognitive dissonance and a strategy to achieve cognitive consistency. Which of the following strategies would most likely achieve cognitive consistency?

    A   Adding new cognitions that are not consistent with pre-existing ones
    B   Changing cognitions involved in the dissonant relationship
    C   Changing the behaviour that is consistent with the cognitions
    D   Gathering new information to substantiate the original beliefs
    E   Holding on to previously held beliefs despite evidence to the contrary

76. Which of the following statements about the Likert scale is correct?

    A   It has a lower sensitivity compared with a dichotomous scale
    B   It is a four-point scale that indicates the level of agreement with presented statements
    C   It is difficult to administer
    D   It leads to the same mean score in different response patterns
    E   Ranking is biased

77. Which of the following theories suggests that, when two beliefs are mutually inconsistent, the one that is less firmly held will change?

   A   Festinger's cognitive dissonance theory
   B   Heider's balance theory
   C   Osgood and Tannenbaum's congruity theory
   D   Post-decision dissonance
   E   Self-evaluation maintenance theory

78. Which of the following theories suggests that people prefer relationships that appear to offer an optimum cost–benefit ratio?

   A   Attribution theory
   B   Equity theory
   C   Proxemics theory
   D   Reinforcement theory
   E   Social exchange theory

DESCRIPTION AND MEASUREMENT

79. Which of the following statements about the Wisconsin card sorting test (WCST) is correct?

   A   It is administered to detect parietal lobe lesions
   B   It consists of 100 cards
   C   It consists of cards that differ solely in terms of colour
   D   It is useful in detecting frontal lobe lesions
   E   The Weschler adult intelligence scale is a part of the WCST

80. Which of the following has the highest life change value according to Holmes and Rahe's social adjustment rating scale?

   A   Birth of a child
   B   Death of a spouse/partner
   C   Divorce
   D   Marriage
   E   Separation from a spouse/partner

81. Which of the following statements is consistent with a selective attention task?

   A   Non-target stimuli are represented among a series of random stimuli on a computer screen
   B   The task is measured by the serial sevens test
   C   The Stroop colour word test assesses selective attention maintained in the face of interference
   D   The target appears on the screen along with randomly distributed target stimuli
   E   The WCST is used to determine selective attention

82. Which of the following statements indicates that a test to measure cognitive function has good construct validity?

   A   The test appears to be good at measuring cognitive function
   B   The test correlates well with other established tests of cognitive function
   C   The test covers most of the important aspects of cognitive function that need to be assessed
   D   The test measures cognitive function accurately
   E   The test produces similar findings when repeated

83. Which of the following statements is consistent with Beck's depression inventory?

    A   It consists of 21 items
    B   It focuses on somatic and behavioural symptoms
    C   It has the highest possible score of 42
    D   It is a clinician-administered scale
    E   It rates symptoms over the last 5 days

BASIC PSYCHOLOGICAL TREATMENTS

84. In cognitive therapy, what does the term 'cognition' refer to?

    A   Attitude
    B   Beliefs
    C   Dissonance
    D   Events
    E   Impairment

85. A 34-year-old depressed man was assessed for cognitive–behavioural therapy. He admitted that he sees things as good or bad, right or wrong. Which of the following cognitive distortions describes this best?

    A   Arbitrary inference
    B   Categorisation
    C   Dichotomous reasoning
    D   Overgeneralisation
    E   Selective abstraction

86. A 54-year-old, married, depressed woman was assessed for cognitive–behavioural therapy (CBT). Which of the following statements about CBT is correct?

    A   It includes optimistic expectation of the future
    B   It includes understanding of the importance of dreams
    C   It suggests that life events play an important part in the genesis of depression
    D   It uses the concept of positive reinforcement
    E   It was influenced by the work of Albert Ellis

87. A 32-year-old woman with agoraphobia was assessed for behaviour therapy. Which of the following is she fearful of?

    A   Family history
    B   Crowds
    C   Heights
    D   Open spaces
    E   Recent life events

88. A 24-year-old man with social anxiety disorder was assessed for behaviour therapy. Which of the following is included in behavioural assessments?

    A   Assimilation
    B   Habituation
    C   Incubation
    D   Preparedness
    E   Resistance

PREVENTION OF PSYCHIATRIC DISORDER

89. A 24-year-old woman had had psychotic symptoms for several months before seeking treatment. Which of the following statements about the duration of an untreated first-episode psychosis (DUP) is correct?

   A   The benefits of reducing the DUP have not been established
   B   The benefits of reducing the DUP appear to be long-lasting
   C   There is no significant difference in the outcome if treated early
   D   Only the negative symptoms of psychosis improve with a short DUP
   E   Only the positive symptoms of psychosis improve with a short DUP

90. An 18-year-old man with sub-threshold symptoms of psychosis is prescribed low-dose risperidone along with CBT. Which of the following statements is correct with regard to the transition to first-episode psychosis after treatment?

   A   Sixty per cent of patients transition to first-episode psychosis
   B   An antipsychotic alone is as effective as combination therapy
   C   Negative symptoms are a strong predictor for transition
   D   The onset of a first-episode psychosis is delayed
   E   There is no effect on the severity of the neurotic symptoms

91. A 60-year-old man with a 30-year history of bipolar affective disorder has been stable on lithium for many years. His serum urea and creatinine levels have recently been steadily increasing above the normal levels. Which of the following is the most appropriate treatment to maintain his current level of stability?

   A   Chlorpromazine
   B   Depot antipsychotics
   C   Lamotrigine
   D   Sodium valproate
   E   Trifluoperazine

92. A 35-year-old woman with a history of recurrent depressive disorder has been stable for a long time on sertraline 100 mg/day. She wishes to conceive and is considering whether or not to taper and stop medication before attempting conception. Which of the following is the most likely scenario if this woman decided to do so?

   A   She has a two-fold risk of relapse
   B   She has a five-fold risk of relapse
   C   She has a ten-fold risk of relapse
   D   She has an approximately 30% increased risk of relapse
   E   She will remain well as women are uniquely protected against depressive relapse during pregnancy

DESCRIPTIVE PSYCHOPATHOLOGY

93. A 74-year-old man is reviewed in the outpatient clinic after a stroke. It is observed that he has severe lability of mood, and involuntary episodes of crying and laughing. What is the most likely psychopathology seen in his case?

   A   Depression
   B   Emotional incontinence
   C   Mania
   D   Mixed affective state
   E   Rapid cycling affective disorder

94. An 80-year-old woman diagnosed with severe depression believes that her intestines have stopped working and her other internal organs are degenerating, suggesting that she is dead and a walking corpse. Which of the following delusions is most appropriate to describe her belief?

A   Grandiose delusions
B   Guilt delusions
C   Infidelity delusions
D   Nihilistic delusions
E   Persecutory delusions

95. A 33-year-old man with schizophrenia takes the offered hand but withdraws it several times without shaking hands. Which of the following symptoms is he exhibiting?

A   Ambitendence
B   Ambivalence
C   Chorea
D   Negativism
E   Stereotypy

96. A 10-year-old boy speaks clearly and fluently in school but becomes mute when at home. Which phenomenon is described in this case?

A   Akinetic mutism
B   Elective mutism
C   Poverty of speech
D   Selective mutism
E   Stammering

97. A 23-year-old man's mother died in an accident. Instead of feeling sad, he laughs and makes jokes with others. Which of the following terms describes this behaviour?

A   Alexithymia
B   Blunted affect
C   Flat affect
D   Incongruent affect
E   Labile affect

98. Which of the following is a formal thought disorder?

A   Delusions of persecution
B   Tangentiality
C   Thought broadcasting
D   Thought insertion
E   Thought withdrawal

99. A 33-year-old woman with an obsessive–compulsive disorder gets intrusive thoughts about the safety of her husband. To cope with these thoughts, she prays three times, buys things in multiples of three and washes her hands three times on each occasion that she experiences these thoughts. Which of the following is most appropriate to describe her behaviour?

A   Compulsions
B   Coping skills
C   Delusions
D   Flight of ideas
E   Normal behaviour

100. A 40-year-old woman feels odd sensations such as electric shocks coming from her feet and that she is having sexual intercourse while asleep. Which of the following is most likely to describe her experience?

    A   Delusions of persecution
    B   Overvalued idea
    C   Passivity phenomenon
    D   Nihilistic delusions
    E   Somatic hallucinations

101. A 22-year-old African man covers his head with a cap. He claims that he is doing this to prevent people from hearing his thoughts, which apparently can be transmitted from his head. What is the most likely description?

    A   Over-valued idea
    B   Thought blocking
    C   Thought broadcasting
    D   Thought echo
    E   Thought insertion

102. A 35-year-old woman believes that Bill Clinton is in love with her. She has never met Bill Clinton. However, she believes that he is posting her love letters through adverts in the newspaper. Which of the following terms is most appropriate to describe her belief?

    A   Capgras' delusion
    B   Cotard's syndrome
    C   Couvade's syndrome
    D   De Clerambault's delusion
    E   Othello's syndrome

103. A 32-year-old woman with a diagnosis of schizophrenia believes that she had a sex change operation at the age of 7 years and since then became a female. Which of the following terms best describes her experience?

    A   Delusional memory
    B   Delusional mood
    C   Depression
    D   Negative symptoms
    E   Positive symptoms

104. An 18-year-old man was recently diagnosed with a first episode of psychosis. He has a sense of perplexity and uncertainty, and feels that something is wrong around him, but can't describe what it is. What is he most likely experiencing?

    A   Delusional memory
    B   Delusional mood
    C   Depression
    D   Negative symptoms
    E   Positive symptoms

105. A 40-year-old man with alcohol dependence saw his wife talking to her boss at work. Since then he believes that she was having an affair with her boss that involved a sexual relationship, despite a lack of evidence. Which of the following is most likely to describe his belief?

    A   Capgras' delusion
    B   Cotard's syndrome
    C   Couvade's syndrome
    D   De Clerambault's delusion
    E   Othello's syndrome

106. An 82-year-old woman believes that her body was infested by parasites. She brought her skin scrapings in a box to the outpatient clinic saying that these were the mites. Which of the following is most likely to explain her presentation?

    A   Capgras' delusion
    B   Cotard's syndrome
    C   Couvade's syndrome
    D   Delusory cleptoparasitosis
    E   Ekbom's syndrome

107. A 19-year-old male student was in a rush to catch the last flight to Poland. In his haste, he read Holland as Poland and reached the wrong terminal. Which of the following terms is most likely to describe his behaviour?

    A   Affect illusion
    B   Completion illusion
    C   Delusion
    D   Hallucination
    E   Pareidolic illusion

108. A 40-year-old woman with a phobia of the dark sees a figure of a 'ghost' when she looks at a tree on a dark night. Which of the following terms is most likely to describe her experience?

    A   Affect illusion
    B   Completion illusion
    C   Delusion
    D   Hallucination
    E   Pareidolic illusion

109. A 7-year-old boy sees the figure of a car when he looks into the clouds. Which of the following terms is most likely to describe his experience?

    A   Affect illusion
    B   Completion illusion
    C   Delusion
    D   Hallucination
    E   Pareidolic illusion

110. A 36-year-old man with a diagnosis of schizophrenia hears the voice of his dead mother whenever he hears the noise of water running from a tap. Which hallucination is most likely being described?

    A   Elementary hallucination
    B   Extracampine hallucination
    C   Functional hallucination
    D   Reflex hallucination
    E   Reverse hallucination

111. A 36-year-old man with a diagnosis of schizophrenia sees different colours in the sky whenever he hears the noise of water running from a tap. Which hallucination is most likely being described?

    A   Elementary hallucination
    B   Extracampine hallucination
    C   Functional hallucination
    D   Reflex hallucination
    E   Reverse hallucination

112. A 40-year-old man with a diagnosis of schizophrenia hears the voice of his dead sister who was buried in another village 30 miles away from his town. Which hallucination is most likely being described?

   A   Elementary hallucination
   B   Extracampine hallucination
   C   Functional hallucination
   D   Reflex hallucination
   E   Reverse hallucination

DYNAMIC PSYCHOPATHOLOGY

113. A 29-year-old male CT3 psychiatric trainee was put down badly by his consultant in a ward round. He wasn't able to say anything to the consultant when the consultant shouted at him. When he returned home, he became verbally abusive and aggressive towards his wife. What is the most likely phenomenon?

   A   Displacement
   B   Identification
   C   Projection
   D   Reaction formation
   E   Regression

114. A 26-year-old male CT1 psychiatric trainee was put down badly by his consultant in a ward round and the consultant shouted at him. After work, he went to see his mother and started to present childish behaviour such as playing with his old toy cars. Which is the most likely defence mechanism?

   A   Displacement
   B   Isolation
   C   Projection
   D   Regression
   E   Sublimation

115. A 27-year-old male CT2 psychiatric trainee was put down by his consultant in a ward round and the consultant shouted at him. After work, he went to the gym and exercised for half an hour more than usual. What is the most likely phenomenon?

   A   Reaction formation
   B   Repression
   C   Sublimation
   D   Turning against self
   E   Undoing

116. A 40-year-old male follower of Mahatma Gandhi does not cooperate with the extra and unnecessary tasks given to him by his manager at work. He never displays his anger by shouting or becoming physically aggressive. What is the most likely phenomenon?

   A   Aggression
   B   Isolation
   C   Passive aggression
   D   Regression
   E   Repression

HISTORY OF PSYCHIATRY

117. In which year was Sigmund Freud born?

   A   1852
   B   1854
   C   1856
   D   1858
   E   1860

118. Where was Sigmund Freud born?

   A   America
   B   Brazil
   C   Czech Republic
   D   Germany
   E   Spain

BASIC ETHICS AND PHILOSOPHY OF PSYCHIATRY

119. The police arrived on your ward and enquired about one of your patients. Under which circumstances would you be able to breach patient confidentiality?

   A   Domestic dispute
   B   Investigation of a serious crime
   C   Participation in riots
   D   Possession of cannabis for personal use
   E   Patient caught shop-lifting

120. Which statement is correct about the consent to participate in clinical research?

   A   All clinical drug trials require adult participants to give informed consent
   B   Consent must be witnessed by someone who is independent and part of the trial team
   C   Consent must be written to be valid
   D   Information sheets for research must refer to the evidence base for the trial
   E   Participants can withdraw consent to all data collected at any time during the study

121. Thought insertion, withdrawal, broadcasting, and delusions of perception and control are all the first rank symptoms of schizophrenia. Who first proposed these first rank symptoms?

   A   Carl Schneider
   B   Emil Kraepelin
   C   Eugene Bleuler
   D   Kurt Schneider
   E   Sigmund Freud

122. A 20-year-old man presented with shallow mood and his thoughts were disorganised. He was diagnosed with hebephrenic schizophrenia. Who described hebephrenic schizophrenia?

   A   Eugen Bleuler
   B   Emil Kraeplin
   C   Ewald Hecker
   D   Kurt Schneider
   E   William Tuke

123. A 26-year-old male school teacher presents with anhedonia, which is a lack of pleasure in activities that were previously enjoyable. Who is most closely associated with the term 'anhedonia'?

A   Donald Cameron
B   Karl Kahlbaum
C   Jabob Moreno
D   Théodule-Armand Ribot
E   Peter Sifneos

124. A 43-year-old man finds it difficult to verbalise his emotions. His psychiatrist friend says that it is alexithymia. Who is most closely associated with the term 'alexithymia'?

A   Donald Cameron
B   Karl Kahlbaum
C   Jabob Moreno
D   Théodule-Armand Ribot
E   Peter Sifneos

STIGMA AND CULTURE

125. Which of the following is seen in latah?

A   It is a dissociative state
B   It is an acute paranoid state that occurs after use of street marijuana
C   It is closely associated with religion
D   It is usually found in South America
E   It is treatable by 'suggestibility'

126. Which of the following is consistent with Da Costa's syndrome?

A   It is a culture-bound syndrome found in North America
B   It is closely associated with depression
C   It is treatable by aspirin
D   Syncope is a prominent symptom
E   Symptoms are similar to those of cardiac dysfunction

127. Susto is also translated as 'fright sickness'. Which statement about susto is correct?

A   It is a depressive state
B   It is a psychotic state
C   It is an obsessive state
D   It is seen in North America
E   It responds to antidepressants

128. When severe, which of the following conditions is called espanto?

A   Brain-fag syndrome
B   Da Costa's syndrome
C   Latah
D   Susto
E   Windigo

129. Windigo is a culture-bound syndrome. Which statement about windigo is correct?

A   It is classified as a culture-bound psychotic syndrome in the DSM-IV
B   It is the compulsive desire to become a cannibal
C   It is found in South America
D   It is treated by an antipsychotic drug
E   It presents mainly with anxiety symptoms

130. Brain fag is a culture-bound syndrome. Which statement is regarding brain fag is correct?

A   It causes the patient to have difficulty in remembering and concentrating
B   It is a condition of fading brain in elderly people
C   It is a psychotic disorder
D   It occurs as a result of eating infected animal's brains
E   It presents with symptoms that occur in the form of tiredness all over the body

Answers: MCQs

1. E Three-word recall

Patients with severe depression can present with significant cognitive impairment such as poor concentration and short-term memory problems. Cognitive functions can be clinically evaluated by performing an MMSE. In this test, three-word recall is used to test short-term memory. Drawing intersecting pentagons, naming, repetition, a three-stage command, reading and writing are useful for testing language. Tests of serial sevens and spelling backwards are used to evaluate attention and concentration. In addition, the MMSE includes tests for orientation to time and place. The clock-drawing test is used to screen executive functions, and visuospatial and constructional praxis. It is not a part of the MMSE, although it is usually used alongside this test.

2. E Perseveration is a sign of a frontal lobe lesion

Perseveration occurs when mental operations persist beyond the point at which they are relevant. This includes senseless repetition of words, gestures or actions. Perseveration is related to the severity of the task facing the patient. It is common in generalised and focal organic brain disorders. For a person with a frontal lobe lesion, the ability to plan ahead is impaired or lost. Other signs and symptoms of frontal lobe dysfunction include cognitive difficulties such as poor short-term memory, poor working memory and impairment of executive functions, behavioural difficulties such as utilisation, aggression, increased sexuality and emotional difficulties. Agnosis is related to receptive aphasias in which the patient experiences sensory stimuli but cannot recognise objects. Dyscalculia is a specific learning disability involving difficulties with calculations.

3. A Attention

The MMSE is a brief structured interview designed to assess cognitive status. It provides quantitative measurements of orientation, memory, calculations and other aspects of the systematic mental state examination. The maximum score is 30 points. The test of serial sevens tests attention and concentration. Registration and recall tests immediate and short-term memory respectively.

4. D The muscle tone is preserved

Automatism is defined as a state that occurs during an ictal or post-ictal state and is characterised by clouding of consciousness. In this state, muscle tone and posture are preserved, though there may be limited awareness of action. It lasts from a few minutes to several hours and the individual may have little to no recollection of events. Automatism can be used as a defence in a criminal case. The legal definition of automatism is an act committed during a state of unconsciousness or grossly impaired consciousness. Such an act lacks a guilty mind. There are two types of automatisms: sane and insane. The difference between the two is based on whether the automatism or behaviour leading to the offence is likely to recur. Sane automatisms are considered singular events resulting from exogenous causes, such as confusional states, hypoglycaemia or night terrors. They lead to a full acquittal. Insane automatisms are viewed as events caused by a disease of the mind that are likely to recur. They therefore require control of the individual to ensure public safety and can lead to a verdict of not guilty by reason of insanity.

5. B Amnesia of the episode

Ganser's syndrome was first described in 1898 when it was indentified in four criminals. It is characterised by approximate answers, clouding of consciousness, auditory or visual hallucinations, and amnesia of the episode. Perseveration, echolalia, echopraxia and hysterical paralysis may be observed. Interestingly, these symptoms are worse when the patient is being observed. It is associated with a recent history of head injury or severe emotional stress, and may be followed by depression.

6. D Delirium

In this clinical scenario, patient has fluctuating consciousness, impaired concentration and cognitive impairment that suggest that he has delirium. There is no evidence of psychotic symptoms or panic disorder. The overdose might have been precipitated by stress or an argument with the patient's girlfriend. An adjustment disorder is not associated with cognitive impairment.

7. D Non-fluent expressive dysphasia

The clinical features in this case scenario indicate that the patient has frontal lobe dementia. A lesion in the left frontal lobe can result in Broca's aphasia which is characterised by reduced frequency of speech and relatively preserved comprehension. Language is reduced to a few disjointed words and the failure to construct sentences. Left temporoparietal damage results in language that is fluent although the words themselves are incorrect. This is known as Wernicke's aphasia, receptive aphasia or posterior aphasia. Dysarthria simply means disordered articulation, i.e. slurred speech. Dyslexia describes a delayed and disorganised ability to read and write.

8. E Vascular dementia

Initially, the term 'catastrophic reaction' was applied to a patient's performance on neuropsychological assessment. A catastrophic reaction manifests as disruptive emotional behaviour when a patient is given a difficult task. It occurs especially when a patient is unable to solve a problem. The damage to the language areas plays an important part in its aetiology. It is commonly seen in Alzheimer's disease, vascular dementias and stroke.

9. D The trail-making test

Working memory and attention can be assessed by the trail-making test. This test includes 2 parts and involves accurately joining 25 dots as fast as possible. The behavioural inattention test (BIT) is a test for detecting and measuring the severity of visual neglect, primarily in stroke and head-injured patients. It consists of six conventional tests which include star cancellation and line cancellation. It also includes nine behavioural tests. The Hayling and Brixton tests assess aspects of frontal executive functions. The Hayling sentence completion test measures the ability to inhibit a habitual or prepotent response. The Brixton test measures the ability to detect rules in sequences of stimuli and concept formation. The token test helps to measure auditory comprehension in patients with aphasia due to stroke. The zoo map is a test of planning.

10. D Matrix reasoning

The Wechsler adult intelligence scale has both verbal and performance components. The verbal IQ is tested using subtests such as similarities, vocabulary, information, arithmetic, digit span and comprehension. The performance IQ is calculated based on picture completion, digit symbol coding, block design, matrix reasoning and picture arrangement. Symbol search, letter–number sequencing and object assembly are other subtests.

11. D Remote

In this case, the situation tests remote memory, which is recollection of past events. Working memory and immediate memory last for seconds. Recent memory is for a few hours at most. Procedural memory is more implicit, e.g. driving a car.

12. B 2

The Glasgow coma scale is useful in assessing and monitoring a patient's level of consciousness. It is classified into best motor response, best verbal response and best eye-opening response. The eye-opening response is scored as follows: 1 = not opening the eyes, 2 = opening eyes to pain, 3 = opening the eyes to speech and 4 = spontaneously opening the eyes.

13. D Raven's progressive matrices

This consists of a series of visuospatial problem-solving tasks, which are thought to tap general intelligence, i.e. they are relatively independent of educational or cultural background. Test–re-test reliability is > 0.8 and internal reliability is > 0.7. It has a published normative rate-of-decay profile, which is defined as the normal pattern of failing more items as the test becomes progressively more difficult. This allows the detection of individuals who are faking poor performance, e.g. in compensation claims. The California verbal learning test is used to test verbal memory. The national adult reading test is used to test premorbid intelligence in English-speaking individuals with dementia. The Cambridge contextual reading test is used to measure premorbid intelligence in individuals with mild-to-moderate dementia. It has a higher predictive value than the national adult reading test. The WAIS is used to measure intelligence in adults and adolescents.

14. E Vascular dementia

NINDS-AIREN (NINDS–AIREN = Neuroepidemiology Branch of the National Institute of Neurological Disorders and Stroke–Association International pour la Recherche et l'Enseignement en Neurosciences) criteria are useful in the diagnosis of vascular dementia.

NINCDS/ADRDA (NINCDS/ADRDA = National Institute of Neurological and Communicative Diseases and Stroke/Alzheimer's Disease and Related Disorders Association) criteria are useful in the diagnosis of Alzheimer's dementia.

The international consensus criteria for dementia with Lewy bodies are used for the diagnosis of Lewy body dementia.

The Lund–Manchester criteria and NINDS criteria are useful for the diagnosis of frontotemporal dementia. Normal pressure hydrocephalus is characterised by a triad of symptoms: ataxia, dementia and urinary incontinence

15. D Matrix reasoning

The verbal IQ is calculated based on the sum of subtests: vocabulary, similarities, arithmetic, digit span, information and comprehension. Factor analysis has suggested that these subtests do not fall neatly into verbal and performance IQ; instead four factors emerge: verbal comprehension, perceptual organisation, working memory and processing speed. With the addition of three further subtests (symbol search, letter–number, sequencing and object assembly), it is also possible to calculate the scores on these four factors. The WAIS-III is a significant improvement on its predecessors in terms of better norms, improved artwork for visually presented items, and reliability coefficients for IQ scales and indices (0.88–0.97).

16. D When light shone back to the left eye from the right, the pupil dilates

Relative afferent pupillary defect (RAPD) occurs when there has been incomplete damage to the afferent pupillary pathway; this can occur with retrobulbar neuritis. Complete recovery may be apparent, but RAPD is still detected on routine examination. This deficit is detected using the swinging-flashlight test. In this case, when light is shone in the left affected eye, it causes both pupils to constrict. The light is swung to the right eye and both pupils constrict and then it is swung back to the left affected eye and the pupil dilates. This clinical observation indicates that there is incomplete damage in the afferent pupillary pathway.

17. D Pure word deafness

This is a syndrome of isolated loss of auditory comprehension and repetition, without any abnormality of speech, naming, reading, or writing. Auditory sound agnosia is a similar syndrome in which the individual is unable to hear nonverbal sounds, e.g. the sound of a bell ringing, despite having intact hearing.

18. B Optic chiasma

Bilateral defects are caused by lesions of the optic chiasma, and include pituitary neoplasms, meningiomas, craniopharyngiomas and secondary neoplasms. When one half of the field is affected, it is called hemianopia; when a quadrant is affected, it is called quadrantanopia. Visual field defects caused by lesions of each optic tract, optic radiation and cortex are called 'homonymous' to indicate the different, i.e. bilateral, origins of each unilateral pathway.

19. D Toxoplasma encephalitis

Patients who are HIV positive and have acquired immune deficiency syndrome are prone to opportunistic infections. Toxoplasmosis is the most common opportunistic infection in the brain in this group of patients. *Toxoplasma gondii* causes encephalitis and cerebral abscess, usually because of reactivation of previously acquired infection. It is treated with pyrimethamine combined with sulfadiazine and folinic acid.

20. A Abnormal synacthen test

In this case, the patient has Addison's disease (primary hypoadrenalism), which is characterised by weight loss, anorexia, malaise, weakness, depression, nausea, vomiting, diarrhoea, myalgia and pigmentation (dust, slaty grey–brown). The short tetracosactide (synacthen) test is indicated for a diagnosis of Addison's disease and screening for adrenocorticotropic hormone (ACTH) deficiency should also be carried out. A patient with Addison's disease will show an impaired cortisol response to ACTH (normal response: 30-min cortisol >600 nmol/L). A patient with Addison's disease will have hypokalaemia. Acanthosis is a diffuse hyperplasia with thickening of the stratum spinosum. A low level of ceruloplasmin is seen in Wilson's disease.

21. D Increased free serum copper

The clinical presentation described is consistent with a diagnosis of Wilson's disease, also known as hepatolenticular degeneration. It is a rare autosomal recessive disorder due to a defect in the Wilson's disease gene (*ATP7B*) located on chromosome 13. It is characterised by deposition of copper in various parts of the body, including the liver, basal ganglia and cornea. In this disorder, free serum copper and 24-hour urinary copper are increased, whereas serum ceruloplasmin and total copper are decreased. A liver biopsy usually indicates increased copper deposition. Treatment includes long-term use of copper-chelating agents such as penicillamine or trientine, a low-copper diet and avoiding food with a high copper content such as chocolate and peanuts.

22. E Raised urinary catecholamine

In this case signs and symptoms indicate that the patient suffers from a phaeochromocytoma. Phaeochromocytomas are tumours of the sympathetic nervous system. They are very rare, with fewer than 1 in 1000 cases of hypertension. Of these tumours 90% arise in the adrenal gland and 10% occur elsewhere in the sympathetic chain; 25% are multiple and 10% malignant. The clinical features are those of catecholamine excess and are frequently, but not necessarily, intermittent. The measurement of urinary metabolites (metanephrines and vanillylmandelic acid) is a useful screening test.

23. A General health questionnaire

Mental disorders in primary care settings pose a considerable burden, not only to the individual and their family but also to primary care services and, economically, to society. The general health questionnaire is designed for use as a screening instrument in primary care, general medical practice or community surveys. There is also a version with subscales for somatic symptoms, anxiety, insomnia, depression and social dysfunction. The other tests are not useful in assessing mood in the given case and presentation in primary care.

24. E Mini-mental state examination

There are numerous tests available to detect cognitive impairment. The MMSE remains a common screening tool for dementia. It is scored out of 30 points and assesses the areas of orientation, registration, recall, language, construction ability, attention and concentration. The clinical dementia rating scale gives an overall severity rating in dementia. The clock-drawing test helps to understand a patient's constructional abilities and, more importantly, his or her planning and organisational ability. Hachinski's ischaemia score helps to differentiate between vascular dementia and Alzheimer's disease.

25. E Wisconsin card sorting test (WCST)

This measures the ability to alter a cognitive set, show deficits in executive and conceptual functions, as well as initiate and monitor the patient's own actions. Some researchers have queried the task's sensitivity to frontal lobe pathology.

26. D Ophthalmoplegia

Wernicke's encephalopathy is classically characterised by the triad of ophthalmoplegia, ataxia and global confusion. Other features may include hypothermia, hypotension, coma, cardiovascular problems and peripheral neuropathies. There is a mortality rate of 10–20% despite adequate treatment.

27. B Anterograde amnesia

Korsakoff's syndrome is characterised by a severe memory defect, particularly for recent events and new information, and the patient compensates for this by confabulation. Polyneuropathy may be present and other associated symptoms may include delirium, confusion, disorientation in time and place, impaired attention and concentration, anxiety fear, depression and delusions. It is caused by thiamine deficiency.

28. B Calmly leave the interview room

It is important to allow the patient, as far as possible, to describe his symptoms spontaneously. However, when the patient threatens violence it is difficult to follow the current plan of interviewing. It is safer to leave the interview room and obtain further assistance.

29. E Overdose when alone in a hotel room

Suicide increases as a function of age. It is rare in children aged < 12 years. It increases after puberty and the incidence continues to increase in the adolescent years. Adverse life events, especially interpersonal relationship difficulties, unemployment, socio-economic adversity, intention and careful planning are associated with a higher suicide risk.

30. E Transketolase

Transketolase deficiency affects carbohydrate metabolism in the brain and is believed to predispose to the occurrence of alcoholic organic brain complications. Guanylyl cyclase and phospholipase A_2 are examples of effectors for neurotransmitter ligands acting through G-protein couple receptors. Conversion of ethanol to acetaldehyde requires the enzyme alcohol dehydrogenase. Acetaldehyde dehydrogenase deficiency affects alcohol metabolism, resulting in an accumulation of acetaldehyde. This can cause the alcohol flush reaction.

31. E Poor parental supervision

Causes of juvenile delinquency are complex and overlap with the causes of conduct disorder. They include social factors (e.g. low social class, poverty, poor housing and poor education), family factors (e.g. large family size, child-rearing practices including erratic discipline, harsh or neglecting care, martial disharmony, inconsistent and ineffective discipline, parental violence and aggression) and child factors (e.g. low IQ, educational and reading difficulties).

32. C Functional abnormalities in the prefrontal area

Attention deficit hyperactivity disorder is an aetiologically heterogeneous disorder, with genetic, neurochemical, affective–cognitive and social environment adversities contributing to the overall liability for the disorder. Genetic studies indicate heritability estimates of 70% or more. Neuroimaging studies show functional abnormalities in the prefrontal area, and other areas associated with executive function and the cerebellum.

33. E Ventral tegmental area dopamine and enkephalin

Availability of alcohol is a powerful determinant of the level of consumption. Culture and tradition are potent influences on the pattern of drinking. The start of drinking is influenced by the setting, the company and expectancies about the likely effects. A number of biological markers have been identified that may predict a vulnerability to developing alcohol abuse. They include reduced electroencephalography α activity and reduced P300 wave amplitude.

34. B Antisocial behaviour

Conduct disorders in childhood consist of temper tantrums, oppositional behaviour, irritability, aggression, stealing, lying, bullying and truancy. Continuation into adult life is common and over 50% of patients will have problems as adults.

35. A Being born in an urban area

The risk factors for developing schizophrenia are family history, migrant or ethnic minority status, chronic cannabis or stimulant use, urban birth or residence, obstetric complications, maternal flu, malnutrition and winter birth. Genetic studies suggest that environmental factors contributing to the aetiology of schizophrenia are more likely to be unique or non-shared rather than familial.

36. A Charles Bonnet syndrome

The Charles Bonnet syndrome is a syndrome of visual hallucinations without any other psychotic symptoms or any evidence of mental illness. It consists of formed, complex, persistent, repetitive and stereotyped visual hallucinations. The patient recognises them as unreal, which may be enjoyable or distressing. This condition is associated with visual impairment.

37. B Delirium

The cardinal feature of delirium is disturbed consciousness with disorientation in time and place, which typically fluctuates over the course of 24 hours with nocturnal deterioration. Two broad patterns of presentation are recognised. One pattern is where the patient is restless, irritable and over-sensitive to stimuli with psychotic symptoms and the other pattern is where there is psychomotor retardation and perseveration without psychotic symptoms.

38. A Acute stress reaction

In this case, signs and symptoms are suggestive of an acute stress reaction. It shares one of the two main criteria for post-traumatic stress disorder, which is the presence of a traumatic event. It starts within minutes of a traumatic event. The acute stress reaction resolves within hours in the absence of a stimulus and in 1–3 days in the presence of a stimulus. The resolution of symptoms starts in 8 hours in the absence of a stimulus and in 48 hours in the presence of a stimulus.

39. E Post-traumatic stress disorder

In this case, signs and symptoms are suggestive of post-traumatic stress disorder. After exposure to a traumatic event, this condition can occur within 6 months and, in certain instances, beyond this period. The symptoms include avoidance of the place of the incident, reliving the incident repeatedly, nightmares, irritability, hypervigilance and an exaggerated startled response. Patients can have an inability to recall certain parts of the incident.

40. D Other neurotic disorders

According to the ICD-10 classification system, neurasthenia is classified under other neurotic disorders. There are two main types of neurasthenia. In one of the types, affected individuals complain of increased tiredness after minimum mental effort and have disturbances in their concentration and thought processes. In the other type of neurasthenia, affected individuals present with physical symptoms such as weakness and tiredness. They complain of aches, pains and muscle weakness. In addition, neurasthenia can present with irritable mood, lack of interest and sleep disturbance.

41. D More user friendly than the DSM-IV

The ICD-10 classification system is clinically–oriented and less rigid in its definitions. It is less suitable for research purposes. Owing to its clinical orientation, the ICD-10 is more user–friendly than the DSM-IV. On the other hand, the DSM-IV is operational and has rigid definitions. It is suitable for research purposes. The ICD-10 is published by World Health Organization and is used widely in the UK and other parts of Europe. The DSM-IV is published by the American Psychiatric Association and is used widely in the USA.

42. C Personality disorder is classified on a separate axis in the DSM-IV

The DSM-IV and ICD-10 are two of the most widely used psychiatric classification systems. Personality disorder is classified separately on axis II in the DSM-IV, whereas in the ICD-10 it is classified along with current mental state diagnosis. The ICD-10 classification system does not distinguish between bipolar I and bipolar II since it was recognised after the ICD-10 was published in 1992. Recurrent brief depressive disorder is a new addition to the ICD-10. Schizotypal disorder is classified with schizophrenia in the ICD-10, whereas it is classified with personality disorder in DSM-IV. Borderline personality disorder, as found in the DSM-IV, is classified as an emotionally unstable personality disorder in the ICD-10.

43. D The ICD-10 was developed by the World Health Organization whereas the DSM-IV was developed by the American Psychiatric Association

The ICD-10 is available in all widely spoken languages. It has a single axis in chapter V. However, a separate, three-axis, multiaxial ICD-10 classification is available for use. The DSM-IV is available in English only and is a five-axis, multiaxial system. The ICD-10 has different versions for research, clinical work and primary care, whereas the DSM-IV has only one version. The ICD-10 does not include social consequences of clinical disorders, unlike the DSM-IV.

44. B Global assessment of functioning

The five-axis classification in the DSM-IV was designed to provide information on a patient's clinical disorder and level of functioning. The axes are as follows:

Axis I: clinical disorders

Axis II: personality disorders, mental retardation

Axis III: general medical condition

Axis IV: psychosocial and environmental problems

Axis V: global assessment of functioning

45. D There is 95% protein binding

Benzodiazepines have a weak organic basis, so when they are subjected to physiological buffering they become lipid soluble to varying degrees – from moderate to high. Absorption from the gastrointestinal tract is complete and followed by first-pass metabolism. Diazepam and flurazepam are among the most rapidly absorbed compounds, with almost complete bioavailability after oral administration. Their kinetics conform to a two-compartment model, with the plasma concentration curve reflecting distribution and metabolism. Desmethyldiazepam is an active metabolite that undergoes slow oxidation before excretion, and therefore has a very long half-life of 30–100 hours. Food reduces the rate, but not the extent, of absorption of diazepam. Diazepam's elimination half-life in young adults and elderly people is 20 hours and 30–100 hours respectively.

46. C The dexamethasone suppression test is mostly unaffected

Benzodiazepines have perhaps the highest therapeutic index of all psychotropic drugs and are extremely effective. It is therefore sometimes problematic to understand whether the 'side effects' represent adverse effects. The dexamethasone suppression test is largely unaffected in benzodiazepine use. However, in chronic high-dose therapy, benzodiazepines may interfere with the dexamethasone suppression test. In therapeutic doses, they have little effect on the cardiovascular and respiratory systems, although sometimes they can cause respiratory depression and reduce systolic blood pressure. Benzodiazepines inhibit the afferent pathways in the spinal cord, resulting in skeletal muscle relaxation. Neuroendrocrine systems are generally unchanged but occasionally plasma cortisol may be reduced.

47. B The concentration of an intravenously administered drug declines exponentially

The elimination of most drugs follows exponential or first-order kinetics, i.e. a constant fraction of the whole drug in the body is eliminated per unit of time. This corresponds to an exponential decline in concentration. The rate of absorption depends on the dose remaining to be absorbed. The rate of elimination depends directly on the amount of drug remaining in the body. The metabolism of alcohol in human beings follows zero-order kinetics. This means that the rate of absorption is independent of the concentration, i.e. the amount metabolised is fixed rather than the proportion of the drug. Bioavailability is the extent to which the drug reaches the systemic circulation when taken by a patient orally or parentally, compared with the same dose of drug given intravenously. Bioequivalence is dependent on efficacy, which in turn depends on plasma concentration.

48. D Naproxen

Fluvoxamine, when used with naproxen, increases the risk of bleeding. In addition, it should be used with caution when given together with lithium (or non-steroidal anti-inflammatory drugs [NSAIDs]), St John's wort, tryptophan or warfarin. Fluvoxamine inhibits the cytochrome P450 CYPIA2/2CG/3A4.

49. D Neuroleptic malignant syndrome

The patient has developed signs of the neuroleptic malignant syndrome. This is characterised by hyperthermia, rigidity, confusion and autonomic lability. It has a reported mortality rate of 20% and it can result in residual neurological deficits in survivors. The neuroleptic malignant syndrome usually resolves on discontinuation of the implicated antipsychotic and medical measures such as rehydration, correction of electrolytes and benzodiazepines if necessary. Dantrolene is another medication that can be used if necessary.

50. C Nausea

One of the common side effects of acamprosate is nausea. Other side effects include diarrhoea, abdominal pain, fluctuations in libido, pruritus and maculopapular rash. Acamprosate is a γ-aminobutyric acid agonist and glutamate antagonist. It is useful in maintaining abstinence in patients with strong cravings for alcohol. It should be started as soon as abstinence has been achieved, and continued for at least one year for optimum benefit.

51. D 5-HT$_{2A}$ receptors increase glutamate release

5-Hydroxytryptamine (5-HT$_{2A}$) receptors excite cortical pyramidal neurons, increase glutamate and decrease dopamine release. These receptors are involved in the mechanism of sleep and hallucinations. Blockade of 5-HT$_{2A}$ receptors leads to release of dopamine. 5-HT$_2$A antagonism decreases extrapyramidal side effects.

52. B α$_2$

All but one of the adrenergic receptors are postsynaptic. The only presynaptic adrenergic receptor is the α$_2$- receptor. This is also known as apresynaptic autoreceptor. It is a G-protein couple receptor.

53. D Stimulation of α$_1$- receptors leads to serotonin release

Noradrenaline and serotonin neurons control each other in the central nervous system. Noradrenaline can control serotonin release both positively and negatively, i.e. stimulation of α$_1$- receptor leads to release of serotonin, whereas stimulation of presynaptic α$_2$- autoreceptors lead to inhibition of serotonin release (feedback inhibition). On the other hand, serotonin has only A negative feedback inhibitory role on noradrenaline release, through. stimulation of 5-HT$_{2A}$- or 5-HT$_{2C}$ -receptors.

54. D α$_2$-Receptor antagonism

Mirtazepine is classified as a noradrenergic and selective serotonergic antidepressant. It is an antagonist of presynaptic α$_2$- adrenergic receptors, thus facilitating serotonin release. It acts as an antagonist of many other receptors including 5-HT$_{2A}$ and 5-HT$_{2C}$.

55. D Serotonin, noradrenaline and dopamine

Venlafaxine has a unique mode of action. In low doses it acts on the serotonin system only. As the dose increases it acts on noradrenergic as well as serotonergic neurons. At higher does, i.e. 225 mg or above, it acts on all the three neurotransmitters, i.e. serotonin, noradrenaline and dopamine. In a nutshell, venlafaxine blocks the serotonin, noradrenaline and dopamine reuptake. In addition blocking noradrenaline reuptake in the frontal cortex could increase dopamine neurotransmission in this part of brain.

56. B Buspirone

Buspirone is an anxiolytic medication with 5-hydroxytryptamine (5-HT$_{1A}$) partial agonist activity. It is a potent D$_2$-receptor antagonist. It is mainly used for treatment of generalised anxiety disorder and other anxiety disorders. Even though it is an antianxiety medication, it is not related to benzodiazepines or barbiturates. It is not helpful for treating benzodiazepine withdrawal symptoms. These patients will need benzodiazepines to relieve their symptoms before starting buspirone.

57. D Haloperidol

High-potency neuroleptics such as haloperidol, pimozide and trifluoperazine have potent tic-suppressing effects. The usual dose of haloperidol is 1–8 mg. Newer antipsychotics such as risperidone and olanzapine have also been used for treatment of Gilles de la Tourette's syndrome with limited success. Risperidone is usually used in a dose range of 1–6 mg.

58. D Figure–ground differentiation

Gestalt psychology is primarily concerned with perceptual processes. It maintains that aspects of perception reflect the brain's innate capacity to order simple sensations in characteristic ways. It holds that the whole or total quality of the image is perceived. According to gestalt psychology, the organisation of stimuli into the image is based on laws of perception, which include:

- Similarity (similar images are grouped together even when separated physically)
- Proximity (nearer images are grouped)
- Closure (gaps are filled into complete a shape)
- Good continuation (images that appear to continue in the same direction are grouped)
- Common fate (images that are more together in a scene are grouped)
- Reversible figures (such as the Necker cube)
- Object constancy (despite expectations)
- Perceptual set

59. D Preoperational stage

This description refers to the concept of egocentrism which is not merely selfishness. It is the restricted ability of a child to view the world from a single point of view which develops at age 2–7 years. This was demonstrated using the mountain task, in which a child would not be able to say what the other person could see from the other side of the desk when only one side of the mountain toy was shown to the child.

60. B Formal operational stage

Hypothetico-deductive reasoning develops in a proportion of children after the age of 12 years. It is characterised by manipulation of ideas and propositions and reasoning is based on construction of verbal arguments.

61. B Circular reaction

Circular reaction is seen during the sensorimotor stage of Piaget's stages of cognitive development; it develops at age 0–2 years. In this stage, infants develop an ability to recognise that they can make things happen. During the sensori motor stage, an infant's mental efforts are mainly focused on sensory experiences such as vision, hearing and touch. During this developmental stage, language starts to develop and thoughts start to dominate action.

62. D Preconventional morality

In this case, the 8-year-old boy is going through the preconventional morality stage of development.

Kohlberg's theory of moral development is characterised by three levels and six stages, as follows:

Level 1: It is preconventional morality that contains two stages:

Stage 1: Punishment and obedience orientation
Stage 2: Egotistical orientation

Level 2: It is conventional morality that contains two stages

Stage 3: Maintaining good interpersonal relationship, being a good person
Stage 4: Maintaining social law and order

Level 3: It is postconventional morality that contains two stages

Stage 5: Social contract or legalistic orientation
Stage 6: Universal principle of justice

63. A Conventional morality

In this case, the 6-year-old boy is going through the conventional morality development stage. Kohlberg's theory of model development is characterised by three levels and six stages.

Level 2 is conventional morality that contains two stages: maintaining good interpersonal relationships, being a good person and maintaining social law and order. They believe that what pleases others is right, so they try to avoid disapproval and to meet the expectations of others.

64. C 12 months

The child is able to say one word such as mummy, doggie. Hence, his age is likely to be 12 months. The following indicates speech development and corresponding age group:

- 6 months (4–10 months): at this age child starts babbling
- 9 months: child starts babbling repetitively
- 12 months: child says words like mamma, papa. This is called the one-word stage
- 24 months: child says 'mamma come'. This is called the two-word stage

65. A 3 years

As a child grows, the fear of darkness develops at age 2–3 years, a fear of supernatural things at 5–8 years and a fear of bodily injury and disasters is seen from age 9–12 years. From age 0–6 months, a fear of falling and of loud noises is evident. Fear of strangers develops at the age of 1 year.

66. E 9 months

A child can hold his head up at age 3 months. He does oral exploration at age 5 months. At age 6 months, palmar grasp develops. By age 9 months the child can sit unsupported and pickup objects with a pincer grasp.

67. C 3–5 years

There are eight Erickson's stages of psychosocial development. In this example, the child is going through the initiative versus guilt stage which is seen between 3 years and 5 years.

Erikson's stages of psychosocial development:

1. Trust versus basic mistrust: birth to 18 months
2. Autonomy versus shame: 18 months to 3 years
3. Initiative versus guilt: 3–5 years
4. Industry versus inferiority: 6–12 years
5. Identity versus role confusion: adolescence
6. Intimacy versus isolation: young adulthood
7. Generativity versus stagnation: middle adulthood
8. Ego integrity versus despair: late adulthood

68. B Anxious avoidant

This is an example of anxious avoidant attachment pattern. Mary Ainsworth has described four main types of attachment on the basis of a strange situation procedure. A secure type of attachment is seen in 65% of infants. In this case, the infant uses the caregiver as a secure base, explores freely, may or may not be distressed at separation, but greets positively on reunion, seeks comfort, settles down and returns to exploration. Anxious avoidant attachment is seen in 20% of infants. In this case the infant appears normally interested in the caregiver, explores busily, minimal distress at separation, and ignores or avoids caregiver on reunion. Resistant/Ambivalent attachment is seen in 10% of infants. In this case there is minimal exploration, and the infant stays closer to the carer, and both seeks and resists contact on reunion. Disorganised attachment is seen in 15% of infants. In this case the infant is disorganised and presents with disoriented behaviour, such as freezing or odd postures, in the presence of the caregiver.

69. B Oral phase

The oral phase of Freud's psychosexual development is seen between 0 and 18 months. Object constancy is Margaret Mahler's sixth subphase and lasts from 2 years to 5 years. Stranger anxiety occurs from 7 months till the end of the first year. Separation anxiety develops at age < 1 year. It peaks between 9 and 18 months and diminishes by about 2.5 years of age. Piaget's sensori motor stage is from 0 years to 2 years. The conventional morality stage of Kohlberg is between 7 and 12 years.

Mahler's developmental phases are:

- Normal autism (0–2 months)
- Symbiosis (2–5 months)
- Differentiation (5–10 months)
- Practising (10–18 months)
- Rapprochement (18–24 months)
- Object constancy (2–5 years)

70. D Temperament

Thomas and Chess conceptualised temperament as representing the behavioural style in children. In the 30-year-long New York Longitudinal Study nine categories of dimensions were observed (e.g. activity level, adaptability, mood) and temperament was categorised into three main types:

1. Easy temperament: 40%

2. Difficult temperament: 10%

3. Slow to warm up: 15%

Rest ungrouped: 35%

Attachment: John Bowlby; object constancy: Margaret Mahler; and imprinting: Lorenz

71. C Egocentric thinking

A characteristic feature of the sensorimotor stage (before 2 years) is a lack of object permanence. This is similar to the situation of 'out of sight out of mind'. Other stages include primary, secondary and tertiary circular reactions. Animistic thinking (inanimate objects seen as being alive) and egocentric thinking (being unable to consider the world from any viewpoint other than their own) are a part of the preoperational stage. Conservation and transitive inference are mastered in the concrete operational stage. Conservation means an understanding that the quantity or amount of a substance or group of objects remains unchanged when nothing has been added or taken away from it.

72. A Each stage is a prerequisite for the next stage of development

Each stage is a prerequisite for one of the four stages of cognitive development described by Jean Piaget (sensorimotor, preoperational, concrete operations and formal operations). These stages lead to capacity for an adult's thought. Each stage is a prerequisite for the next one.

73. D Social learning incorporates both classic and operant models

There are three types of learning: classic, operant or instrumental, and social learning which incorporates classic and operant conditioning. Classic conditioning is a result of environmental events whereas operant learning is thought to result from the consequences of a person's actions. Learning is defined as the change in behaviour resulting from repeated practice; both the environment and the behaviour interact to produce the learned change.

74. B Classic conditioning is the association of a neutral stimulus with a conditioned stimulus which brings a response originally elicited by an unconditioned stimulus

In classic conditioning, there is pairing of a conditioned or neutral stimulus with an unconditioned stimulus (response), such that the neutral stimulus eventually evokes an unconditioned stimulus. In habituation, response to repeated stimuli decreases and eventually disappears over time. Instrumental and operant learning are one and the same. Social learning occurs by observations, identification and role modelling.

75. B Changing cognitions involved in the dissonant relationship

Cognitive dissonance refers to the discomfort produced by inconsistent cognitions. It is therefore an unpleasant feeling caused by having simultaneous conflicting ideas. Cognitive consistency can be achieved by changing attitudes, beliefs and actions. The way in which a person thinks is called cognition and cognition affects a person's behaviour. Cognitive dissonance occurs when a person holds simultaneous conflicting ideas, e.g. if a person fails an exam, he says that even the better candidates didn't pass; by doing this he reduces their dissonance. In the classic example of *The Fox and the Grapes* by Aesop, the fox sees grapes hanging up high and has a strong desire to eat them. However, the fox is unable to reach them and so thinks that the grapes are not worth eating as they must be unripe or sour. The fox reduces his dissonance by denigrating the value of the grapes (this is where the expression 'sour grapes' comes from).

76. D It leads to the same mean score in different response patterns

The Likert scale is a five-point scale indicating the level of agreement with presented statements. It has several advantages including its increased sensitivity compared with the dichotomous Thurstone scale. It is more easily administered. A disadvantage is that the response patterns may result in the same mean score.

77. C Osgood and Tannenbaum's congruity theory

Osgood and Tannenbaum's congruity theory suggests that, when two beliefs are mutually inconsistent, the one that is less firm will change. It is oriented to communication and persuasion. Festinger's cognitive dissonance theory suggests that, when an individual's behaviour is inconsistent with his or her attitude, it leads to dissonance, which in turn leads to change of attitude so that it is consistent with the behaviour. Fritz Heider's balance theory is that individuals seek harmony of attitudes and beliefs and they evaluate related things in a similar manner. Self-evaluation maintenance theory suggests that the skills or interests that define us can cause dissonance when they appear to be superior in others close to us. Postdecision dissonance is where one justifies an unalterable decision as the right one.

78. E Social exchange theory

Social exchange theory suggests that people prefer relationships that appear to offer an optimum cost–benefit attraction. It also involves comparison of various attractive options. This theory is influenced by other disciplines such as economics, sociology and psychology. According to equity theory, the cost–benefit of a relationship for each person is approximately equal in a preferred relationship. Reciprocal reinforcement explains the attraction that occurs with rewards in both directions. Proxemics relate to the interpersonal space body buffer zone.

79. D Is useful in detecting frontal lobe lesions

The WCST is used to test set-shifting ability, which is thought to be a function of the frontal lobe. It consists of a pack of cards, each of which has a number of coloured shapes. There are three possible shapes, three possible colours, and one, two or three exemplars of the shape that could appear on each card. The patient has to sort the pack of cards into three piles, but is given no instructions as to the sorting principle.

80. B Death of a spouse/partner

Life events have emerged as risk factors for the onset of major depression, suicide and other psychiatric morbidity. They are given weighting that relates to the closeness of the lost relative and the impact on the individual patient. Their impact depends on the individual's personality and genetic endowment.

81. A Non-target stimuli are represented among a series of random stimuli on a computer screen

Selective attention, i.e. focused attention, involves a mechanism by which certain information is registered and other information rejected, whether or not the latter enters conscious awareness. The cocktail party phenomenon is an example in which we manage to select one or two voices to listen to from the hubbub of conversation taking place in the same room. In the Stroop colour word test, the patient is asked to name the colour in which the words are written; if the words are unrelated to colour, the colour of the print is compatible with meaning. Thus, in the Stroop test, there is competition between the automatic and the controlled processing systems.

82. B The test correlates well with other established tests of cognitive function

Construct validity refers to whether a test measures a specified and well-defined construct, e.g. if a test measures cognitive function there should not be clusters of items from other aspects of the mental state.

83. A Consists of 21 items

Beck's depression inventory (BDI) is a 21-question, self-rating inventory. It is sensitive to change, but is biased towards cognitive items. It can be used in children aged > 13 years and adults. The BDI has a copyright and requires permission from the authors for its use.

84. D Events

Cognitive therapy emphasises how the patient comes to think about him or herself, the future and the world. The cognitive view assumes that one assigns meaning and value to one's perceptions and experiences. Cognitive schemata are organised representations of prior experiences that help a person to screen, encode and categorise perceptions. Cognitive therapy is primarily concerned with cognitive events.

85. C Dichotomous reasoning

Cognitive therapy is more than the routine application of a series of techniques. The focus is on the cognitive factors that maintain emotional disturbance and maladaptive behaviour. Dichotomous reasoning means that the person sees things in black and white. Arbitrary inference means that the person jumps to conclusions despite contradictory or insubstantial evidence. Overgeneralisation refers to when a single incident is accepted as an invariable rule or consequence. Selective abstraction means that the person takes a detail out of context and misses the significance of the whole situation.

86. E It was influenced by the work of Albert Ellis

Cognitive–behavioural therapy refers to a method of therapy based on a theory of emotional disorders. Theoretically, the emphasis is on information processing, i.e. individuals react, feel and behave according to how they process the information contained in the environment. Albert Ellis had named it in rational–emotive therapy.

87. B Crowds

Agoraphobia is anxiety associated with places or situations either from which escape may be difficult or in which help may not be available in the event of a panic attack. It means literally fear of the crowded place. It is strongly associated with panic.

88. D Preparedness

Behavioural therapy assumes that a person's behaviour is a way of adapting to the environment, and not necessarily a reflection of some kind of underlying psychopathology. Preparedness is an inherited biological trait. It means that things feared may be or have been potentially dangerous to the human race.

89. B The benefits of reducing the DUP appear to be long-lasting

Evidence suggests that treatment of the first episode of psychosis with an aim of a shorter duration of untreated psychosis (DUP) results in improved positive and negative symptoms of psychosis. In addition, treatment with an emphasis on a shorter DUP is associated with significantly improved social functioning compared with a longer DUP. Early intervention in psychosis is based on multimodal treatment, such as antipsychotic medications, psychology and social aspects of care. As per the available evidence, the advantages seem to be permanent rather than temporary.

90. D Onset of a first episode of psychosis is delayed

A randomised controlled trial, conducted at the personal assessment and crisis evaluation clinic (PACE clinic) in Melbourne, concluded that cognitive therapy alone or in combination with a low-dose antipsychotic can delay the onset and reduce the severity of the first episode of psychosis in patients with sub-threshold symptoms. In addition to reducing the severity of psychotic symptoms, there is a reduction in non-psychotic symptoms and distress following treatment. However, monotherapy with an antipsychotic was not as efficacious as cognitive therapy alone or in combination. The transition to the first episode of psychosis is strongly associated with the presence of positive symptoms.

91. D Sodium valproate

Of the given options, sodium valproate is effective in the prophylaxis of bipolar affective disorder. The National Institute for Health and Care Excellence (NICE) recommends sodium valproate as a first-line option for the treatment of acute manic episodes, in combination with an antidepressant for the treatment of depressive episodes and for prophylaxis. Lithium is a effective medication in treating acute manic episode and also effective in the prophylaxis of bipolar affective disorder. Most of the side effects are dose related. Common side effects are nausea, vomiting, gastrointestinal upset and tremors. It can cause a person to drink more and pass more urine. It can also reduce the capacity of the kidneys to concentrate urine: it reduces the glomerular filtration rate. Lithium can cause interstitial nephritis in a small number of patients. The risk of relapse may be reduced by decreasing the dose gradually over a period of at least a month and avoiding incremental serum reductions of >0.2 mmol/L.

92. B She has a five-fold risk of relapse

It is now well established that stopping antidepressants soon after treatment is associated with a high risk of relapse. Controlled studies involving patients with recurrent depression have shown that maintenance treatment with antidepressants can substantially reduce relapse rate.

93. B Emotional incontinence

In this case, after a stroke the patient has developed emotional incontinence. It is a neurological sign when an affected individual is unable to control laughter and/or crying. It is characterised by sudden onset of laughter or crying episodes which last for a few seconds to minutes, and can occur several times a day. It is an extreme form of labile affect. It is also known as a pseudo-bulbar affect. This sign is observed in patients with brain injury, frontal lobe damange, stroke, multiple sclerosis and other neurological illnesses. In this case, there are no signs and symptoms to suggest depression and bipolar disorder.

94. D Nihilistic delusions

This case description is an example of Cotard's syndrome in which the patient presents with nihilistic delusions that she is dead and her internal organs are degenerating or have stopped working. This condition is found in patients with psychotic depression and schizophrenia. In grandiose delusions patients believe beyond doubt that they possess special powers and abilities. In delusions of guilt, patients have inappropriate and extreme feelings of guilt which are not based in reality. In persecutory delusions, the most common delusions, patients believe that they are being followed, persecuted or spied upon. In delusions of infidelity, also known as morbid jealousy, patients are convinced that their partner has been unfaithful contrary to evidence suggesting otherwise.

95. A Ambitendence

In this scenario, the patient has ambitendence which is characterised by a state of cooperation and opposition (take the offered hand and withdraw), leading to incompletion of the task (hand shake). It is one of the catatonic signs observed in schizophrenia. Another catatonic sign is negativism, in which a patient will resist or oppose all passive movements. Stereotypy is an extensive repetition of movement, speech pattern, ideas or posture, which could be simple or complex in nature. Chorea is the abnormal and involuntary movements seen in neurological disorders such as Huntington's disease, Sydenham's chorea and Wilson's disease. Ambivalence is a state in which an individual experiences both positive and negative feelings towards a person or thing.

96. D Selective mutism

Elective mutism was a term used in the DSM-III to describe refusal to speak in all social situations despite a normal ability to interact. However, this was redefined in the DSM-IV as a refusal to speak in specific situations despite normal ability and termed 'selective mutism'. This form of mutism is seen in children with emotional or psychiatric disorder. It is also seen in adults with hysteria, depression, schizophrenia or organic disorders. Akinetic mutism is usually seen in frontal lobe injury, when a person refuses to move and speak. Poverty speech is an inability to initiate or participate in a conversation, and speech usually lacks content that is not prompted. In stammering, the normal flow of speech is interrupted.

97. D Incongruent affect

Affect is a pattern of observable behaviour, that is an expression of feelings or emotions. It is variable over time and changes in response to changing emotional state. In this case description, the observed affect (laughs and jokes) is different to subjective affect (sadness); it is termed 'inappropriate affect'. Maintenance of an affective state is termed 'stability of affect'. Labile affect in the absence of such stability can be seen as a sudden unprovoked change in affect in which patients can cry or laugh excessively for no apparent reason. The inability to express emotions is termed 'flat affect', whereas restricted ability to express emotions is termed 'blunt affect'. Alexithymia is an inability to recognise and use words to describe emotions and feelings.

98. B Tangentiality

A formal thought disorder is considered to be a schizophrenic language disorder characterised by disordered speech, and results from disorganised thoughts. It is often a symptom of schizophrenia, mania, severe depression with psychosis and other psychotic disorders. Tangentiality is a formal thought disorder in which there is tangential association of ideas leading to disruption in the smooth continuity of speech. Knight's move thinking, drivelling, omission, derailment and circumstantiality are other examples of formal thought disorders. Thought insertion, thought broadcasting, thought withdrawal and thought block are Schneider's first rank symptoms. Delusion of presecution is a fixed belief in which patients believe that they are being followed, persecuted and spied on, and that the perceived persecutor will cause them harm.

99. A Compulsions

Obsessions are repetitive, senseless, intrusive thoughts that are recognised as irrational thoughts by the sufferer. Several unsuccessful attempts have been made to resist these thoughts. The content of the thought can be related to aggression, dirt, contamination, fear of causing harm, and religious or sexual thoughts. In order to reduce the associated anxiety symptoms patients carry out repetitive acts such as counting, cleaning repeatedly, or touching or arranging things in symmetry; these acts are termed 'compulsions'.

100. E Somatic hallucinations

Perceptual disturbance such as hallucinations are false sensory perception in the absence of external stimulus. Hallucinations can be mood congruent or mood incongruent. These can be auditory, visual, gustatory, olfactory and somatic in nature. Somatic hallucinations can be tactile or haptic which involves either superficial sensations or sensations just under the skin in the absence of real stimulus.

101. C Thought broadcasting

Thought insertion, thought withdrawal; thought broadcasting and thought echo are Schneider's first rank symptoms of schizophrenia. In addition, delusion of perception, delusion of control and 3rd person auditory hallucinations is other first rank symptoms (though not Schneiderian). In thought broadcasting, the patient believes that their thoughts are being broadcasted and people are aware of what they are thinking.

102. D De Clerambault's delusion

Another term for De Clerambault's syndrome is erotomania. In this condition, the patient believes that an exalted or well-known person is in love with him or her. In Cotard's syndrome, the person believes that he or she is dead or some part of his or her body is rotten or doesn't exist. Couvade's syndrome is an abnormality of experience of self, in which a spouse/partner complains of obstetric symptoms during his partner's pregnancy. In Capgras' syndrome, the patient believes that someone close has been replaced by an exact double. Othello's syndrome, also known as morbid jealousy – a condition in which an individual believes that his or her spouse or partner is unfaithful.

103. A Delusional memory

Delusional mood, delusional perception, delusional memory and sudden delusional ideas constitute primary delusions. Delusional memory is a condition in which, even though in reality something has never happened, the individual believes and reports an irrational or false event as if it had occurred in the past. In delusional mood, a person senses that there is a change in the environment but is unable to make sense of this change, resulting in being perplexed. In delusional perception, a patient gives new meaning to normally perceived objects.

104. B Delusional mood

Delusional mood, delusional perception, delusional memory and sudden delusional ideas constitute primary delusions. In delusional mood a person thinks that there is something wrong around him but he doesn't know what is wrong. Positive symptoms of schizophrenia comprise delusions and hallucinations, whereas negative symptoms of schizophrenia consist of apathy, poverty of speech, and blunted and incongruent affect.

105. E Othello's syndrome

Othello's syndrome is also known as morbid jealousy. In this condition, an individual believes that his or her spouse or partner is unfaithful. De Clerambault's syndrome, also known as erotomania, is a condition in which that patient believes that an exalted or well-known person is in love with him or her. In Cotard's syndrome, the person believes that he or she is dead or some part of his or her body is rotten or doesn't exist. Couvade's syndrome is an abnormality of experience of self, in which a male spouse also complains of obstetric symptoms during his female partner's pregnancy. In Capgras' syndrome, the patient believes that a person who is close has been replaced by an exact double.

106. E Ekbom's syndrome

Delusional parasitosis, aslo known as Ekbom's syndrome is a condition in which an individual develops a delusion, a false belief, that he or she is infested by parasites. Individuals with this condition usually present to specialists such as dermatologists and pest control experts rather than a psychiatrist. Individuals can bring scrapings of their skin or related samples to prove that there are parasites crawling under or on their skin. Delusory cleoparasitosis is a related condition in which the individual believes that the house is infested by parasites rather than the body.

107. B Completion illusion

Hallucinations and illusions are perceptual abnormalities. In an illusion, a stimulus is present but a different object or image is perceived. In a hallucination, the perception occurs in the absence of a stimulus. In a completion illusion, a stimulus that doesn't form a complete object may be perceived as complete. It occurs due to inattention and disappears when an individual concentrates on the object. In this example, because of inattention, the student read Holland as Poland.

108. A Affect illusion

In illusions, a stimulus is present but a different object or image is perceived. In hallucinations, perception occurs in the absence of a stimulus. In completion illusion, a stimulus that doesn't form a complete object may be perceived as complete. Affect illusion arises in the context of a particular mood state. As in this example, due to fear of the dark, the woman sees the figure of a ghost in a tree on a dark night. This disappears on additional concentration.

109. E Pareidolic illusion

In this example, the individual has a pareidolic illusion. In this illusion, which is often playful, the object is formed from ambiguous stimuli and intensifies on additional attention. One such example is seeing figures of cars or human faces when looking into the clouds.

110. C Functional hallucination

In functional hallucinations, an external stimulus provokes the hallucination but the stimulus and hallucination are in same modality as in this case; it is a sound that is perceived individually. Elementary hallucinations are not fully formed. They could be in the form of noises.

111. D Reflex hallucination

Elementary hallucinations are not fully formed. They could be in the form of noises. In functional hallucinations an external stimulus provokes the hallucination but the stimulus and hallucination are in the same modality; in this case it is a sound that is perceived individually. In extracampine hallucinations, the patient has hallucinations that are well beyond the limits of his sensory fields. In reflex hallucination, a person experiences the stimulus in one modality but perceives it in a different modality. In this case the patient sees colours whenever he hears the sound of running water.

112. B Extracampine hallucination

In functional hallucinations, an external stimulus provokes a hallucination but the stimulus and hallucination are in same modality; in this case it is a sound that is perceived individually. In extracampine hallucinations, the patient has hallucinations that are well beyond the limits of his sensory fields. In this case, patient hears the voice of his dead sister far away from his sensory field.

113. A Displacement

Anna Freud described 10 defence mechanisms in her work. Reaction formation, projection and regression are three of them. In displacement, emotions or wishes are transferred from the original object or person to a more suitable substitute.

Reaction formation is seen in patients with obsessive–compulsive disorder. Here the attitude is opposed to the oppressed wish and constitutes the opposite reaction.

Projection: unacceptable thoughts, emotions and feelings are projected on to some other person.

Regression: at the time of stress or threat a person returns to an earlier stage of maturational functioning.

Identification: a person takes the attributes of others to him- or herself.

114. D Regression

Regression is the defence that refers to the reversion to the early stage of ego functioning. Each and every person has defences to deal with stress. Some of them are mature defences such as altruism, sublimation, suppression and humour. Some are immature and neurotic defences such as displacement, isolation regression and projection.

Isolation: thoughts, emotions or behaviour is isolated to break the link with other thoughts or memories.

115. C Sublimation

This is the transformation of our instinctual energy to a more socially acceptable one. So, in this case, rather than shouting back at the consultant, the trainee went to the gym and transformed his anger and frustration into exercising. This is a mature defence mechanism.

116. C Passive aggression

Regression is the defence that refers to the reversion to the early stage of ego functioning, or at the time of stress or threat a person returns to an earlier stage of maturational functioning.

Repression is a type of basic defence in which unacceptable or uncomfortable ideas, thoughts or emotions are pushed away into unconsciousness.

Passive aggression is characterised by non-cooperation with no display of anger.

117. C 1856

Sigmund Freud was born on 6 May 1856. He was born in a town called Moravia, which is now part of the Czech Republic. His father was a wool merchant. He specialised in neurology. When he was in France, he trained in hypnosis. He also worked with hysterical patients, and while working with these patients he developed psychoanalysis.

118. C Czech Republic

Sigmund Freud was born on 6 May 1856. He was born in a town called Moravia, which is now part of the Czech Republic. His father was a wool merchant. He specialised in neurology. When he was in France, he trained in hypnosis. He also worked with hysterical patients, and while working with these patients, he developed psychoanalysis.

119. B Investigation of a serious crime

Although priests and lawyers enjoy their relationships with their clients who preserve the hermetically sealed notion of confidentiality, doctors do not. An unwelcome consequence of the Tarasoff case is to extend the psychiatrist's role as an agent of social control and to give clinicians barriers to predicting dangerousness that they simply do not possess. Respecting confidentiality is only one among an ever-growing list of duties that the doctor must balance against each other.

120. E Participants can withdraw consent to all data collected at any time during the study

The law with regard to consent to medical treatment makes it clear that any unconsented touching of patients by a doctor may be both a civil wrong (tort) and a criminal act (battery). Whether implicit or explicit, the patient's consent will not be valid unless he is informed, capable and free from duress. The doctor is required to impart sufficient, understandable and relevant information to the patient to enable a choice based on the patient's own judgement of the alternatives.

121. D Kurt Schneider

Schneider proposed first rank symptoms of schizophrenia. These are neither diagnostic nor prognostic but indicate schizophrenia. The first rank symptoms are thought insertion, thought withdrawal, thought broadcasting, delusions of perception, passivity phenomena, third person auditory hallucinations and running commentary. The term 'schizophrenia' was coined by Eugene Bleuler in 1911. Carl Schneider described different forms of formal thought disorders.

122. C Ewald Hecker

Hebephrenic schizophrenia is a type of schizophrenia in which affective changes are prominent. The mood is shallow and inappropriate, and thoughts are disorganised. The onset is usually in adolescence. Hecker described hebephrenic schizophrenia. Bleuler coined the term. William Tuke promoted moral treatment for psychiatric patients.

123. D Théodule-Armand Ribot

Anhedonia is lack of pleasure in doing activities that were previously enjoyable. Ribot coined the term 'anhedonia'. Sifneos coined the term 'alexithymia', which is difficulty in verbalising emotions. Moreno is considered to be the father of psychodrama. Kahlbaum described cyclothymia, which is persistent instability of mood, involving periods of depression and mild elation; none of these periods is severe or prolonged enough to fulfil the diagnosis of bipolar affective disorder.

124. E Peter Sifneos

Sifneos coined the term 'alexithymia', which is difficulty in verbalising emotions. It is also described as an inability or difficulty in describing or being aware of one's emotions or mood. It is seen in conditions such as depression, substance misuse or post-traumatic stress disorder.

125. A It is a dissociative state

Latah is a dissociative state triggered by a sudden shock or fright. The patient goes into repetitive speech (echolalia) or movements (echopraxia). This syndrome is most prevalent among middle-aged Malaysian women.

126. E Symptoms are similar to those of cardiac dysfunction

The World Health Organization, in the ICD-10, classifies this condition as a psychosomatic disorder (f 45.30). Also known as 'soldier's heart' it was described by Jacob Mendes Da Costa during the American civil war.

127. A It is a depressive state

Susto is a cultural syndrome condition common to Latin America; it occurs after a sudden traumatic and shocking life event. It is believed that the soul is lost from the body after a traumatic emotional or physical life event, which leads to sadness, sickness and misery. It can be a life-threatening illness and presents with symptoms of lethargy, lack of motivation, insomnia and diarrhoea.

128. D Susto

Espanto is the more severe form of the condition susto (the soul leaves the body due to the individual being frightened by a ghost). The only treatment of susto/espanto is via spiritual means, which includes ritual cleansings, herbs by a *curandero*, a spiritual healer (or *curandera* if female). Women seem to be affected more than men. It is associated with a higher mortality rate compared with the general population.

129. B It is a compulsive desire to become a cannibal

Windigo is a culture-bound syndrome found in Algonquian, which is a Native American tribe. The person has an intense craving for human flesh and there is a compulsive desire to become a cannibal. The person is very scared that he may become a cannibal (windigo monster). It usually occurs during the winter and when food is scarce. It rarely responds to any medication, and is not included in the DSM-IV.

130. A It causes the patient to have difficulty in remembering and concentrating

The origin of this condition is West Africa. Brain fag is usually seen in high school/university students when they are stressed by challenges at university or school. Students will often mention that their brains are 'fatigued' and they cannot concentrate or remember, and have difficulty thinking. Somatic symptoms are centred on the head and neck: pain, pressure, blurring of vision and feelings of heat and burning due to 'too much thinking'. It can resemble certain anxiety, somatoform and depressive disorders.

Chapter 2

Test questions: 2

Questions: MCQs

For each question, select one answer option.

HISTORY AND MENTAL STATE EXAMINATION

1. Which of the following describes blunting of affect?

   A   Inability to show reactivity of affect
   B   Incongruity of affect
   C   Insensitivity to the subtleties of social intercourse
   D   Limitation in the usual range of emotional responses
   E   Stiffening of affect

2. According to the *International Classification of Disease*, 10th revision (ICD-10), which of the following is a criterion for an adjustment disorder?

   A   The patient continues to function normally
   B   The symptoms must occur within 1 month of an identifiable psychosocial stressor
   C   The symptoms persist longer than 6 months in all types of manifestations
   D   There is a correlation with drug-related problems
   E   The disorder category includes separation anxiety disorder of childhood

3. While administering the mini-mental state examination (MMSE) to a 78-year-old man, he asked you what is being assessed by copying the diagram of interlocking pentagons. What would you say to him?

   A   Attention and concentration
   B   Comprehension
   C   Constructional praxis
   D   Copying skills
   E   Geometrical ability

4. Over a period of 18 months, a 41-year-old man developed clumsiness, unsteady gait and poverty of speech. He appeared apathetic, depressed and paranoid. Which of the following is the most likely diagnosis?

   A   Address test
   B   Benton visual retention test
   C   Digit span
   D   Serial sevens
   E   Spelling 'world' backwards

5.   Which of the following statements is correct with regard to eliciting information from patients?

   A   Closed questions are the least frequent causes of interruption
   B   Most patients are allowed to complete their opening statement
   C   Most patients present their problems in a logical order
   D   Most patients take less than 2 minutes to complete their opening statement
   E   The longer the clinician waited, the less information was elicited

6.   The family of a 41-year-old man was concerned that over the past 18 months he had become clumsy and unsteady while walking. He appeared apathetic, depressed and paranoid. His thoughts have slowed down. Which of the following is the most likely diagnosis?

   A   Alzheimer's disease
   B   Creutzfeldt–Jakob disease
   C   Dementia with Lewy bodies
   D   Huntington's disease
   E   Vascular dementia

7.   Which of the following is an example of an open question?

   A   Has your sleep been poor recently?
   B   Have you been feeling depressed recently?
   C   Have you lost any weight recently?
   D   Have you lost pleasures in things recently?
   E   How have you been feeling in your spirits recently?

COGNITIVE ASSESSMENT

8.   Which of the following cognitive functions is assessed by the serial sevens test?

   A   Concentration
   B   Counting
   C   Language
   D   Orientation
   E   Recall

9.   Which of the following is the most accurate statement about the use of the MMSE in the assessment of a patient with suspected dementia?

   A   A score of <23 is diagnostic of Alzheimer's disease
   B   An average patient with untreated Alzheimer's disease will lose 3–4 points per year
   C   MMSE has a high sensitivity for detecting language difficulties
   D   Persevering on items that the patient finds difficult usually gives the best results
   E   The scores correlate highly with detailed neuropsychological tests

10.   A 78-year-old man was brought to the accident and emergency department after being found wandering about during the night. During his assessment, which of the following will help the clinician to distinguish between delirium and dementia?

   A   Disorientation to place
   B   Disorientation to time
   C   Impaired consciousness
   D   Inability to remember three objects
   E   Irritability

11. Most of the neuropsychological tests do not allow one to guess. Which of the following test results is based on how much a patient can actually guess?

    A   Cognitive estimates test
    B   Graded naming test
    C   Paced auditory serial addition test
    D   Pyramids and palm trees test
    E   Stop signal task

12. What is the 'map search' test used to assess?

    A   Attention and concentration
    B   Intelligence
    C   Speed of processing information
    D   The visuospatial ability of a person
    E   Visual memory

13. Which part of the brain is assessed by the trail-making test?

    A   Frontal lobes
    B   Left parietal lobe
    C   Occipital lobe
    D   Right parietal lobe
    E   Temporal lobe

14. Which of the following statements about cognitive dysfunction in schizophrenia is correct?

    A   All individuals who develop schizophrenia have a cognitive dysfunction
    B   Impaired cognitive test performance in patients with schizophrenia is an epiphenomenon
    C   Low IQ at a young age is a risk factor for schizophrenia
    D   Schizophrenia does not cause intellectual decline
    E   Visuospatial memory functioning is a predictor of functional outcome in schizophrenia

15. Which of the following is a feature of the amnestic syndrome?

    A   Impaired intelligence
    B   Impaired procedural memory
    C   Impaired semantic memory
    D   Intact immediate memory
    E   Loss of memory of the period before the brain damage

16. Which of the following neuropsychological tests is found to be accurate in differentiating Alzheimer's disease from depressive pseudodementia?

    A   Addenbrooke's cognitive examination
    B   Clock-drawing test
    C   MMSE
    D   Paired associative learning test
    E   Wechsler adult intelligence scale

NEUROLOGICAL EXAMINATION

17. A 38-year-old man complained of an inability to see in the upper left corner of his vision. On examination, you found a visual field defect in the left upper quadrant of both eyes. Where is the lesion likely to be located in the brain?

    A   Left temporal lobe

B   Pituitary gland
C   Right parietal lobe
D   Right occipital lobe
E   Right temporal lobe

18. A 30-year-old woman gave a history of intermittent numbness, tingling in her limbs and visual impairment. On eye examination, you noticed that, on attempted left lateral gaze, the right eye failed to adduct and the left eye developed coarse nystagmus in abduction. What is the most likely reason for this abnormality of eye movement?

A   Left cranial nerve VI palsy
B   Left internuclear ophthalmoplegia
C   Optic neuritis
D   Right cranial nerve III palsy
E   Right internuclear ophthalmoplegia

19. Your consultant has informed you that a patient who was recently assessed has Bell's palsy, with a lesion in the petrous temporal bone. Which of the following clinical features would indicate the origin of the lesion?

A   Corneal ulceration on the affected side
B   Failure of conjugate lateral gaze (towards the lesion)
C   Hyperacusis
D   Loss of taste on the posterior third of the tongue
E   Normal furrowing of the brow on the same side as the lesion

20. You examined a patient with multi-infarct dementia. From your examination findings, you concluded that he had developed pseudobulbar palsy. Which of the following is consistent with this diagnosis?

A   Emotional stability
B   Fasciculation of tongue
C   Gag reflex lost
D   Reduced jaw jerk
E   Dysarthria

ASSESSMENT

21. A 76-year-old woman complained of mild memory loss, mental and physical slowing, and difficulty in thinking for the past 6 months. On examination, she has a broad-based shuffling gait and a diagnosis of normal pressure hydrocephalus is considered. Which of the following features will help you to confirm the diagnosis?

A   Acalulia
B   Anterograde amnesia
C   Apathy
D   Ophthalmoplegia
E   Urinary incontinence

22. A 25-year-old man with epilepsy and a mild learning disability is brought to the accident and emergency department with aggressive behaviour; he has also been found wandering on the street. He is taking carbamazepine, lithium and zopiclone. Which of the following will help you to understand the possible cause of his presentation?

A   Electroencephalogram
B   Erythrocyte sedimentation rate

C   Full blood count
D   Throat swab
E   Urea and electrolytes

23. A 50-year-old widow is admitted with confusion and aggressive behaviour of recent origin. She is known to have renal failure and depression, for which she takes paroxetine. Which of the following will help you understand the possible cause of her presentation?

A   CT of the brain
B   Erythrocyte sedimentation rate
C   Full blood count
D   Serum paroxetine level
E   Thyroid function tests

24. A 39-year-old man with chronic schizophrenia complained of a sore throat and fever. He was diagnosed as having MRSA (meticillin-resistant *Staphylococcus aureus*) during his previous admission to the medical ward. He had been taking clozapine for the past 2 years. Which of the following will help you understand the possible cause of his current problem?

A   Electroencephalography
B   Erythrocyte sedimentation rate
C   Full blood count
D   Liver function tests
E   Urea and electrolytes

25. An 18-year-old man is considering an application for a university course. However, he has a weak academic record in his school studies. He is regarded as outgoing, level headed, happy and well adjusted, with no previous history of behavioural or emotional difficulties. In response to a referral from his general practitioner, which psychological instrument will be most appropriate in assessing this person?

A   General health questionnaire
B   Halstead–Reitan battery
C   Minnesota multiphasic personality inventory
D   Symptom checklist-90
E   Wechsler adult intelligence scale–revised

26. A 58-year-old chief executive of a National Health Service trust experienced a brief period of mild right-sided paraesthesia and a left-sided headache of 12 hours' duration. After 1 week, he saw his neurologist who observed forgetfulness, decreased understanding of complex information and diminished daily living skills. Which of the following is the most appropriate test in assessing this man?

A   Bender visual–motor gestalt test
B   Halstead–Reitan battery
C   Milton clinical multiaxial inventory
D   Projective drawings
E   Wisconsin card sorting test

27. A 35-year-old single man with a narcissistic personality disorder had received insight-oriented psychotherapy for 1 year. The therapist felt that there was been little or no progress in the therapy for several months. Which of the following tests is most likely to reveal the personality dynamics that might be helpful in understanding the therapeutic impasse?

A   Minnesota multiphasic personality inventory
B   Projective drawings
C   Rorschach's inkblot technique
D   Sixteen personality factors questionnaire
E   Symptom checklist-90

28. Which of the following is a recognised as a poor prognostic factor in anorexia nervosa?

    A   Childhood obesity
    B   Early age of onset
    C   Low social class
    D   Male sex
    E   Poor educational achievement

29. Which of the following is the most common comorbidity associated with a panic disorder?

    A   Agoraphobia
    B   Alcohol misuse
    C   Depression
    D   Drug misuse
    E   Social anxiety disorder

30. A 15-year-old girl presented with a history of dieting and excessive exercising. Her height is 165 cm and current weight 50 kg. What is her body mass index?

    A   Less than 15
    B   Between 16 and 17
    C   More than 20
    D   Between 18 and 19
    E   Below the cut-off to diagnose anorexia nervosa

31. Which of the following is a common neuroendocrine change found in patients with anorexia nervosa?

    A   Decreased corticotrophin-releasing hormone
    B   Decreased plasma cortisol levels
    C   Delayed insulin release
    D   Exaggerated dopamine release
    E   Increased luteinising hormone levels

AETIOLOGY

32. A 21-year-old man informed you that he was a heavy user of cannabis. He was seeking advice about the risks associated with cannabis use. What would you tell him?

    A   Cannabis use can precipitate schizophrenia in people who are vulnerable because of a family history of the disorder
    B   Chronic cannabis use has no effect on motivation and social performance
    C   Long-term cannabis use causes physical dependence
    D   Long-term cannabis use causes severe cognitive impairment
    E   Long-term cannabis use does not cause tolerance

33. Which of the following is the best predictor of long-term general intellectual impairment after a head injury?

    A   Duration of post-traumatic amnesia
    B   Duration of unconsciousness
    C   Glasgow Coma Scale score on admission
    D   Retrograde amnesia
    E   Type of head injury

34. If a person starts smoking cannabis before the age of 15 years, what is the chance of developing a psychotic disorder before the age of 26 years?

   A   Eight times more likely
   B   Four times more likely
   C   Six times more likely
   D   Ten times more likely
   E   Twice as likely

35. What is the prevalence of major depression in older people with congestive cardiac failure compared with cardiac patients with no heart failure?

   A   1:1
   B   1:1.5
   C   1:2
   D   2:1
   E   5:1

36. Which of the following structures is associated with negative symptoms of schizophrenia?

   A   Dorsolateral prefrontal cortex
   B   Hippocampus
   C   Lateral ventricles
   D   Mesolimbic tract
   E   Third ventricle

DIAGNOSIS

37. A 69-year-old retired banker underwent major abdominal surgery. Three days later, he was noticed to be agitated, restless, confused and visually hallucinated. What is the most likely diagnosis?

   A   Delirium tremens
   B   Ekbom's syndrome
   C   Ganser's syndrome
   D   Korsakoff's syndrome
   E   Lewy body dementia

38. A 65-year- old woman presented with a gradual reduction in her verbal fluency, motivation and self-control. She also exhibited a degree of disinhibition. Her EEG was normal. Which of the following best describes her condition?

   A   Alzheimer's disease
   B   Bipolar affective disorder
   C   Depression
   D   Frontotemporal dementia
   E   Multi-infarct dementia

39. Which of the following is not a part of the diagnostic criteria for emotionally unstable personality disorder, according to the ICD-10?

   A   Chronic feeling of emptiness
   B   Involvement in intense and unstable relationships
   C   Recurrent threats or acts of self-harm
   D   Transient stress-related paranoid ideation
   E   Uncertainty about self-image

40. A 21-year-old man was recently reviewed in the emergency department due to an increase in recent bouts of verbal aggression. He did not make any eye contact, continued to talk over the practitioner and was difficult to interrupt. He preferred his own company and had a rigid routine and a keen interest in collecting models of fighter planes. What is the most likely diagnosis?

   A   Attention deficit hyperactivity disorder
   B   Borderline learning disability
   C   High functioning autistic spectrum disorder
   D   Schizoid personality disorder
   E   Schizotypal personality disorder

41. A 19-year-old man was seen in an outpatient clinic after a referral from his general practitioner due to a long-term problem with concentration. On examination, he exhibited an abundance of thoughts which shifted from one task to another and a tendency to act impulsively without thinking through the consequences of his actions. He mentioned that he had lots of energy, his bedroom was in disarray and at work he would stop working on projects once the challenging part was over. He easily became bored with things and did not pay much attention to details. He easily misplaced and lost things. What is the most likely diagnosis?

   A   Asperger's syndrome
   B   Bipolar affective disorder
   C   Borderline personality disorder
   D   Hyperkinetic disorder
   E   No mental disorder

CLASSIFICATION

42. Which pair of clinical features is most likely to be present in persistent delusional disorder?

   A   Bizarre encapsulated delusions and systematised delusions
   B   Blunting of affect and delusions of control
   C   Mood congruent delusions and prominent affective symptoms
   D   Persistent auditory hallucinations and definite evidence of brain disease
   E   Prominent depressive symptoms and persecutory delusions

43. Which of the following statements is characteristic of the ICD-10 diagnostic hierarchy?

   A   Any given diagnosis includes the presence of all the symptoms of higher members of the hierarchy
   B   ICD-9 and ICD-10 have the same hierarchical structure
   C   Neurotic, stress-related and somatoform disorders are in the middle of the hierarchy
   D   Organic disorders are at the bottom of the hierarchy
   E   Schizophrenia and affective disorders are at the same level

44. In some cases of schizophrenia, the ICD-10 allows coding of a fifth character. What does this fifth character signify?

   A   Age of onset of schizophrenia
   B   Duration of schizophrenia
   C   Number of symptoms of schizophrenia
   D   Pattern of course of schizophrenia
   E   Subtype of schizophrenia

45. In the ICD-10, under which category is multiple personality disorder classified?

   A   Dissociative disorder
   B   Enduring personality changes, not attributable to brain damage and disease

C   Habit and impulsive disorder
D   Mixed and other personality disorders
E   Specific personality disorders

46. According to the ICD-10, which of the following categories includes paedophilia?

A   Disorders of sexual preferences
B   Gender identity disorder
C   Habit and impulse control
D   Other disorders such as adult personality and behaviour disorders
E   Psychological and behaviour disorders associated with sexual development and orientation

47. According to the ICD-10, which of the following categories includes the schizotypal disorder?

A   Affective disorders
B   Disorders of psychological development
C   Neurotic, stress-related and somatoform disorders
D   Personality disorders
E   Schizophrenia and related disorders

48. Which of the following is included under schizophrenia in the ICD-10?

A   Disorganised schizophrenia
B   Post-schizophrenic depression
C   Schizoaffective disorder
D   Schizophreniform disorder
E   Schizotypal disorder

49. According to the ICD-10, what is the minimum duration for symptoms of obsession and compulsion to persist in order to meet the criteria of obsessive–compulsive disorder?

A   1 week
B   2 weeks
C   4 weeks
D   6 weeks
E   8 weeks

50. According to the ICD-10, what is the minimum duration of symptoms to meet the criteria for generalised anxiety disorder?

A   1 month
B   2 months
C   6 months
D   1 year
E   2 years

51. In which of the following classification systems is a diagnosis of narcissistic personality disorder included?

A   Both the ICD-10 and the *Diagnostic and Statistical Manual of Mental Disorders*, 4th edn (DSM-IV)
B   DSM-IV only
C   ICD-10 only
D   ICD-9
E   In neither ICD-10 nor DSM-IV

52. What is the duration of symptoms that meets the diagnostic criteria for somatisation disorder in the ICD-10?

A   4 months

    B   6 months
    C   1 year
    D   18 months
    E   2 years

53. What is the duration of symptoms that meets the diagnostic criteria of delusional disorders in the ICD-10?

    A   1 month
    B   2 months
    C   3 months
    D   4 months
    E   6 months

BASIC PSYCHOPHARMACOLOGY

54. Which of the following statements about the properties of trazodone is correct?

    A   It has strong antihistamine properties
    B   It inhibits monoamine oxidase enzymes A and B
    C   It is a 5-hydroxytryptamine (5-HT_2) agonist
    D   It is relatively safe in overdose
    E   It strongly inhibits 5-HT reuptake

55. Which of the following statements about the properties of donepezil is correct?

    A   It blocks the damaging effects of normal excitotoxicity
    B   Its half-life is about 5 hours
    C   It is a carbamate derivative
    D   It is a non-competitive, reversible inhibitor of acetylcholinesterase
    E   It potentiates the action of acetylcholine at the nicotinic receptors

56. You have assessed a 10-year-old boy, with diagnosis of attention deficit hyperactivity disorder, who presents with complaints of severe abdominal pain. He has not taken his medication methylphenidate and clonidine since he ran away from home 2 days ago. He has undergone an extensive physical examination, drug tests and investigations, which proved negative. What is the most likely cause of his abdominal pain?

    A   Clonidine withdrawal
    B   Feigned illness
    C   Independent physical illness
    D   Methylphenidate withdrawal
    E   Psychogenic pain

57. What is the mode of action of atomoxetine in attention deficit hyperactivity disorder?

    A   Calcium channel antagonist
    B   Cholinesterase inhibitor
    C   Dopamine reuptake inhibitor
    D   Noradrenaline reuptake inhibitor
    E   Selective serotonin reuptake inhibitor

58. Which of the following is a triazolopyridine?

    A   Amitriptyline
    B   Amoxapine

C   Diazepam
D   Dothiepen
E   Trazodone

59. Which of the following is a tertiary amine?

A   Amitriptyline
B   Amoxapine
C   Desipramine
D   Nortriptyline
E   Protriptyline

60. Many of the psychotropic drugs can cause priapism. Which of the following is the mechanism for priapism?

A α_1-Receptor agonism
B α_1-Receptor blockade
C α_2-Receptor agonism
D α_2-Receptor blockade
E β_2-Receptor blockade

61. Fluvoxamine is a selective serotonin reuptake inhibitor. Which of the following receptors does it act on to improve cognition and depression?

A   Dopamine-2 receptors
B   Histaminergic receptors
C   Muscarinic receptors
D   Noradrenergic receptors
E   Sigma receptors

62. Which of the following is a risk factor for developing a rash with lamotrigine therapy?

A   Combining it with carbamazepine
B   Combining it with an antipsychotic
C   Exceeding the rate of the recommended dose escalation
D   Being male
E   Being old

63. For the past 2 years, a 42-year-old woman has been prescribed an antiepileptic medication as a mood stabiliser for the treatment of bipolar affective disorder. She has recently developed renal stones. Which antiepileptic drug is likely to have caused this problem?

A   Gabapentin
B   Lamotrigene
C   Tiagabine
D   Topiramate
E   Vigabatrin

64. A 46-year-old woman is prescribed an antiepileptic drug as a mood stabiliser for the treatment of bipolar affective disorder. She complains of tunnel vision. Which of the following is likely to be the drug involved in this side effect?

A   Gabapentin
B   Lamotrigene
C   Tiagabin
D   Topiramate
E   Vigabatrin

65. A 38-year-old man with a history of heroin dependence attended a party and took buprenorphine supplied by a friend. Which of the following symptoms is he most likely to experience?

   A   Bradycardia
   B   Collapse due to opioid overdose
   C   Constricted pupils
   D   Drowsiness
   E   Tachycardia

BASIC PSYCHOLOGICAL PROCESSES

66. A 3-year-old boy was specifically attached to his mother. He became uncomfortable when handled by other members of his family. According to Bowlby, at what age does this specific attachment start to develop in a child?

   A   1–2 months
   B   2–4 months
   C   4–6 months
   D   6–9 months
   E   30–36 months

67. According to the Ainsworth strange situation experiment, a 15-month-old girl plays independently when the mother is nearby but gets distressed when she leaves the room. She then seeks contact with the mother on her return. What type of attachment behaviour is this child exhibiting?

   A   Ambivalent
   B   Avoidant
   C   Disorganised
   D   Resistant
   E   Secure

68. A 30-year-old man gave brief answers or provided positive answers of their experiences without elaborating or explaining. According to Main's semi-structured Adult Attachment Interview, which type of attachment is most likely?

   A   Autonomous
   B   Dismissing
   C   Disorganised
   D   Preoccupied
   E   Secure

69. A 40-year-old woman with a borderline personality disorder became highly emotional when talking about her childhood memories. She often became angry and got distressed for no apparent reason. According to Main's semi-structured Adult Attachment Interview, which type of attachment does she have?

   A   Autonomous
   B   Dismissing
   C   Disorganised
   D   Preoccupied
   E   Secure

70. An infant was studied intensively and followed up at 5, 18 and 22 months. He seemed to adapt poorly to changes, had regular habits and exhibited mild intensity of emotional reactions. According to the New York Longitudinal Study, what type of behaviour does he exhibit?

   A   Difficult

B   Easy
C   Fast
D   Fast to warm up
E   Slow to warm up

71. A 40-year-old man with alcohol dependence presents with short-term memory loss. Which of the following statements describes what is most likely to be absent?

A   Chunking can increase the capacity of short-term memory
B   Short-term memory can be extended by rehearsal
C   Recall of information is error free
D   Short-term memory uses visual coding
E   Short-term memory lasts 15–30 seconds

72. A 75-year-old man remembers everything about his personal history such as the day he was born, the day he got married and the day his first child was born. What type of memory does this describe?

A   Episodic memory
B   Implicit memory
C   Procedural memory
D   Semantic memory
E   Working memory

73. Which of the following statements is untrue for sensory memory?

A   Echoic memory lasts for 2 seconds
B   Iconic memory lasts for 0.5 second
C   If attention is paid, sensory memory enters into short-term memory
D   Sensory memory is modality specific
E   Sensory memory has a short capacity

74. Which of the following is untrue for the mode for retrieval of memory?

A   Recall
B   Recognition
C   Reconstruction
D   Reduction
E   Reintegration

HUMAN PSYCHOLOGICAL DEVELOPMENT

75. Which stage of Piaget's theory of cognitive development is associated with the pendulum experiment?

A   Concrete operational stage
B   Formal operational stage
C   Operational stage
D   Preoperational stage
E   Sensorimotor stage

76. Which of the following statements about Piaget's theory of cognitive development is correct?

A   Castration anxiety is explained in Piaget's cognitive development
B   The concept of conservation and seriation develops during the preoperational stage
C   Deductive reasoning and hypothesis testing develop during the concrete operational stage
D   Egocentrism refers to self-centredness
E   Object permanence is completed at 18 months

77. A 14-year-old boy maintains social order and law and says 'I won't do it because it would break the law'. Which of Kohlberg's stages of moral development does this indicate?

     A   Stage 2
     B   Stage 3
     C   Stage 4
     D   Stage 5
     E   Stage 6

78. Which of the following is associated with the New York Longitudinal Study of Alexander Thomas, Stella Chess and Herbert Birch?

     A   Attachment
     B   Theory of mind
     C   Temperament
     D   Object constancy
     E   Imprinting

79. Which of the following statements about memory is correct?

     A   Memory is divided into short, intermediate and long-term types
     B   Long-term memory is also known as secondary or remote memory
     C   Short- and long-term memory do not differ in the amount of information that can be stored
     D   The capacity of short-term memory is limited 10–15 bits
     E   Working memory and recent memory are synonymous

80. Which of the following is consistent with the concept of cognitive dissonance?

     A   Attribution of an other's behaviour to situational causes
     B   The concept is a cognitive approach
     C   It is concerned with a person changing his or her thinking to lessen harmony
     D   It implies incongruity in a person's beliefs, knowledge and behaviour
     E   It produces a comfortable state

81. Which of the following statements about learned helplessness is correct?

     A   By using this strategy, the individual is able to control events
     B   Learned helplessness is a paradigm used to explain psychosis in depressed individuals
     C   It is learning how to feign helplessness
     D   It teaches an animal how to endure pain in order to avoid an aversive stimulus
     E   The organism learns that no behavioural pattern can influence the environment

SOCIAL PSYCHOLOGY

82. The new Prime Minister was sworn in after a landslide victory. He announced his cabinet soon after a sworn-in ceremony. Which of the following best describes the Prime Minister's social power to choose his cabinet as described by French and Raven?

     A   Authoritative
     B   Coercive
     C   Expert
     D   Referent
     E   Rewarding

83. The teacher strongly believed that the charismatic union leader represented his views at the rally. Which social power, according to French and Raven, is displayed in this case?

    A   Coercive
    B   Informational
    C   Legitimate
    D   Referent
    E   Rewarding

84. What is the view that 'you have of yourself' called?

    A   Ego-self
    B   Integration of the self
    C   Self-concept
    D   Self-esteem
    E   Self-image

85. When measuring an attitude, a scale was used in which there were a large number of statements about a particular issue. Each statement had a numerical value indicating how favourable it could be. People were asked whether they agreed with each of the statements. The total number of 'agree statement' scores was averaged. Which of the following scale is being described?

    A   Borgadus' social distance scale
    B   Likert's scale
    C   Thurtsone's scale
    D   Semantic differential scale
    E   Sociogram

DESCRIPTION AND MEASUREMENT

86. Which of the following can be assessed by a vocabulary test?

    A   Intelligence
    B   Language
    C   Premorbid intelligence
    D   Speech
    E   Visuospatial and perceptual–motor speed

87. Which of the following statements about a diagnostic interview is correct?

    A   An American version of the present state examination (PSE) is called the schedule for affective disorders and schizophrenia (SADS)
    B   PSE can be used to characterise illness
    C   PSE provides no criteria for severity
    D   PSE provides an operational definition of symptoms to be rated
    E   SADS is identical to PSE in its scope of application

88. Which of the following is an observer-rated psychiatric instrument?

    A   Beck's Depression Inventory
    B   General health questionnaire
    C   Leyton's Obsessional Inventory
    D   Present state examination
    E   Severity of alcohol dependence questionnaire

BASIC PSYCHOLOGICAL TREATMENTS

89. A 21-year-old woman university student was assessed for behavioural therapy. Which of the following statements about behavioural therapy is correct?

     A   Analysing life events is an integral part of the process
     B   Associated cognitions cannot be ignored
     C   Concomitant use of a psychotropic drug is necessary
     D   Functional analysis of behaviour is an absolute necessity
     E   Operational definitions are used for behavioural patterns

90. A 28-year-old woman was undergoing behavioural therapy for a phobic disorder. Which of the following statements about the schedule of reinforcement is correct?

     A   A smooth pattern of behaviour is found with a variable-ratio schedule
     B   In a fixed-interval schedule, the rate of the responses increases in direct proportion to the duration of the interval
     C   In a variable-ratio schedule, the rate of the response tends to be slow
     D   'Scalloping' occurs in a variable-interval schedule
     E   The rate of response increase is found with a variable-ratio schedule

91. A 43-year-old male office worker was on sick leave from his work. His doctor had advised him to return to work as soon as possible. However, he was not keen to do so. He was considered to be displaying 'sick role behaviour'. Which of the following statements about this is correct?

     A   It does not allow the patient to be exempted from normal social behaviour
     B   It is an activity adopted by those who consider themselves to be ill
     C   It refers to the effect of the unconscious denial
     D   It refers to the measures taken to detect a disease in the asymptomatic stage
     E   It refers to the measures taken to prevent a disease

92. A 45-year-old woman was assessed for cognitive–behavioural therapy for generalised anxiety disorder. Which of the following statements about the cognitive model of anxiety is correct?

     A   Conditions related to real dangers are responsible for the anxiety
     B   Interpretation of perceived loss is responsible for the anxiety
     C   Life events are responsible for the anxiety
     D   Patient's interpretation of life events is responsible for the anxiety
     E   Patient's responses are appropriate to the situation in which they occur

PREVENTION OF PSYCHIATRIC DISORDER

93. Which of the following was considered to reduce the risk of dementia but is now thought to increase the risk?

     A   Atorvastatin
     B   Donepezil
     C   Hormone replacement therapy
     D   Rivastigmine
     E   Vitamin B_{12}

94. Which of the following options has evidence for delaying the onset of Alzheimer's disease?

     A   Down's syndrome
     B   Drinking small amounts of alcohol

C   Prolonged education
D   Stopping smoking
E   Vitamin supplements

95. Which of the following is a risk factor for relapse into depression during pregnancy?

A   Family history of depression
B   Higher body mass index
C   Higher number of previous depressive episodes
D   Later age of onset of depression
E   Younger age of onset of depression

96. Which of the following statements about Rose's 'preventive paradox' is correct?

A   Preventive measures targeted at high-risk individuals produce the best pay-off for the population
B   Preventive measures targeted at high-risk individuals produce the best pay-off for those individuals
C   Preventive measures targeted at high-risk individuals produce the best pay-off for those individuals, but the best pay-off for the population as a whole is provided by universal measures
D   Universal preventive measures produce the best pay-off for individuals at high risk
E   Universal preventive measures produce the best pay-off for individuals at low risk

DESCRIPTIVE PSYCHOPATHOLOGY

97. You asked a 32-year-old man with schizophrenia to show his tongue and you pricked it with a pin as a part of examination. On asking him to show his tongue again, he puts his tongue out without thinking about the pinprick. How is this phenomenon best described?

A   Advertence
B   Automatic obedience
C   Echopraxia
D   Mannerism
E   Stereotypy

98. A 45-year-old woman visited a place and immediately developed a sense of familiarity because her stored memories were brought into her consciousness. How is this phenomenon best described?

A   Déjà-vu
B   Jamais-vu
C   Recognition
D   Registration
E   Retention

99. Which of the following should not be considered for diagnosis of a delusional disorder?

A   Delusions of control
B   Delusions of infestation
C   Delusions of jealousy
D   Delusions of persecution
E   Hypochondriacal delusions

100. Which of the following is not assessed in the MMSE?

    A   Apraxia
    B   Clock drawing
    C   Reading
    D   Working memory
    E   Writing

101. A 74-year-old depressed woman reported that the antiemetic drug prescribed to her had destroyed her intestines and stopped the blood flowing to her brain. She refused to eat as she believed that she no longer had any bowels. Which of the following phenomena does she describe?

    A   Cotard's syndrome
    B   Couvade's syndrome
    C   Ekbom's syndrome
    D   First rank symptoms
    E   Primary delusions

102. A general practitioner referred a 35-year-old woman to you for an assessment of obsessive–compulsive disorder. Which of the following is the most likely pattern that you would expect in this patient?

    A   A need for symmetry or precision, which leads to a compulsion of slowness
    B   An obsession of doubt, followed by a compulsion of checking
    C   An obsession with dirt or germs, followed by washing or avoidance
    D   Intrusive obsessional thoughts without a compulsion
    E   Magical thinking

103. You have assessed a 65-year-old man in your outpatient clinic. On asking him about the capital of Scotland, he answered Glasgow, on asking about the number of months in a year, he answered 14, and on asking about the colour of an orange, he answered blue. What phenomenon is he most probably displaying?

    A   Confabulation
    B   Cryptamnesia
    C   Dementia
    D   Verbigeration
    E   *Vorbeireden*

104. Which of the following does not explain the process of learning and memory?

    A   Decoding
    B   Encoding
    C   Rehearsal
    D   Retrieval
    E   Storage

105. A 48-year-old man with chronic schizophrenia has been on a stable dose of an antipsychotic drug for 20 years. He came to see you in clinic and frequently made a gesture similar to saluting. What is this phenomenon called?

    A   Mannerism
    B   *Mitmachen*
    C   Stereotypy
    D   Tardive dyskinesia
    E   Tics

106. Which of the following can be conceptualised as the déjà-vu and jamais-vu phenomena?

A   Behaviour
B   Cognition
C   Mood
D   Perception
E   Volition

107. A 27-year-old white woman never left her house without covering her head in a veil. On enquiry into this she told you that she did not want other people to hear what she thought. What is her most likely psychopathology?

A   Third person hallucination
B   Thought broadcasting
C   Thought echo
D   Thought insertion
E   Thought withdrawal

108. Which of the following examples cannot be classified among first rank symptoms of schizophrenia?

A   *Écho de la pensée*
B   Feeling of sunrays directed by US army satellites entering inside the knee, and causing the pain
C   Patient knew that he was the Wimbledon tennis champion when he saw the Wimbledon underground signboard
D   Voices asking the patient to go to London and meet the Queen
E   Voices commenting on the patient's actions

109. A 34-year-old alcohol-dependent man presents to the accident and emergency department due to a distressing sensation of little animals crawling over his body. What is this phenomenon?

A   Delirium tremens
B   Delusion of infestation
C   Haptic hallucination
D   Kinaesthetic hallucination
E   Lilliput's hallucination

110. A 27-year-old woman was in a hurry to catch the last train to Hertford. She was already late. However, in her hurry, she read Hereford as Hertford and boarded the train for Hereford. What is the most likely phenomenon?

A   Affect illusion
B   Completion illusion
C   Imagery
D   Pareidolic illusion
E   Pseudoillusion

111. A 45-year-old male inpatient refused to accept his medication. He said that his doctor is an imposter even though he acknowledged that he looks the same. What psychopathology does he have?

A   Capgras' syndrome
B   Fregoli's syndrome
C   Illusion of doubles
D   Syndrome of intermetamorphosis
E   Syndrome of subjective doubles

112. Which of the following does not explain the process of 'forgetting'?

    A   Decay
    B   Ineffective decoding
    C   Ineffective encoding
    D   Interference
    E   Motivated forgetting

113. A 47-year-old man was observed to be walking sideways along the hospital corridor. When asked for the reason, he said that it was 'because of the side effects'. Which of the following explains this observation?

    A   Adverse effects of his medication
    B   Concrete thinking
    C   Impaired judgement
    D   Loss of ego boundaries
    E   Poor insight

DYNAMIC PSYCHOPATHOLOGY

114. Which of the following is a narcissistic defence mechanism?

    A   Introjection
    B   Projection
    C   Regression
    D   Repression
    E   Schizoid fantasy

115. Which of the following disorders is associated with an ego defence mechanism of avoidance?

    A   Conversion disorder
    B   Depression
    C   Obsessive–compulsive disorder
    D   Post-traumatic stress disorder
    E   Social anxiety disorder

116. What is the reservoir of feelings, thoughts, urges and memory that is outside our conscious awareness known as?

    A   Id
    B   Ego
    C   Ego-ideal
    D   Super-ego
    E   Unconscious

117. Which of the following is a narcissistic defence mechanism?

    A   Acting out
    B   Anticipation
    C   Displacement
    D   Projection
    E   Regression

118. Which of the following statements about a transitional object is correct?

    A   Anna Freud used it to encourage transference in the analysis of children at play
    B   It is commonly used by a child to manage anxiety

C   It is commonly used by people with learning disabilities to manage anxiety
D   It impedes a satisfactory progress of mourning
E   It was a concept first used by Melanie Klein

HISTORY OF PSYCHIATRY

119. A 35-year-old man with schizophrenia presented with waxy flexibility. His psychiatrist diagnosed him as having catatonia. Who coined the term 'catatonia'?

A   Bleuler
B   Hecker
C   Kahlbaum
D   Kraepelin
E   Schneider

120. In the 1960s, patients with schizophrenia improved after treatment with chlorpromazine. Who is associated with the introduction of chlorpromazine?

A   Bleuler
B   Cade
C   Deniker
D   Kahlbaum
E   Kane

121. A 30-year-old man with schizophrenia heard voices commenting on his actions and believed that his actions were controlled by aliens. These are two of the first rank symptoms. Who was the first to propose it?

A   Carl Schneider
B   Emil Kraepelin
C   Eugene Bleuler
D   Kurt Schneider
E   Ross

122. A 24-year-old young woman with a history of prominent mood changes presented with shallow mood, and inappropriate and disorganised thoughts. The onset is usually in adolescence with this type of schizophrenia. Who first described it?

A   Bleuler
B   Griesinger
C   Hecker
D   Schneider
E   Tuke

123. A 35-year-old single man was going through a depressive episode of moderate severity. He mainly lacked interest in his daily activities and hobbies. His psychiatrist said that he had anhedonia. Who coined this term?

A   Cameron
B   Kahlbaum
C   Moreno
D   Ribot
E   Sifneos

124. A 40-year-old man experienced his first episode of bipolar affective disorder–current episode mania. He was assessed by a psychiatrist who observed tangentiality and circumstantiality while speaking and described the symptoms as a formal thought disorder. Who proposed formal thought disorder for the first time?

A   Carl Schneider
B   Emil Kraepelin
C   Eugene Bleuler
D   Kurt Schneider
E   Ross

125. Maslow's triangle represents the hierarchy of needs where, to reach the higher level, the lower level must be satisfied. In which year was this theory put forward?

A   1923
B   1938
C   1943
D   1949
E   1950

126. Which of the following drugs was introduced in 1967 as the first antipsychotic depot injection?

A   Clopixol (zuclopenthixol decanoate)
B   Depixol (flupenthixol decanoate)
C   Haldol (haloperidol decanoate)
D   Modecate (fluphenazine decanoate)
E   Piportil (pipothiazine palmitate)

127. Who discovered the design of randomised controlled trials?

A   Bradford Hill
B   Delay and Deniker
C   John Cade
D   Leonard
E   Paul Janssen

128. Tricyclic antidepressants (TCAs) were discovered long before other antidepressants. Which of the following was the first TCA to be used?

A   Clomipramine
B   Desipramine
C   Imipramine
D   Iproniazid
E   Trimipramine

129. Who is associated with schizoaffective psychosis?

A   Hecker
B   Jasper
C   Kahlbaum
D   Kasanin
E   Schneider

130. Who is associated with the treatment of mania with lithium?

A   Biltz
B   Cade
C   Delay and Deniker
D   Janssen
E   Kane

BASIC ETHICS AND PHILOSOPHY OF PSYCHIATRY

131. Which of the following statements about stigma and mental illness in the Indian subcontinent is false?

    A   The person fears rejection by parents
    B   Men suffer from stigma more often than women do, because they are breadwinners
    C   The person needs to hide the condition from others
    D   Older people are more stigmatised than young people
    E   The stigma was related to fear of job prospects

132. In terms of evidence of prejudice against mental illness, which of the following is correct?

    A   People with mental illness provoke distaste or disgust in others
    B   Most of the public are generally hostile towards people with mental illness
    C   Most of the public resent people with mental illness
    D   There is a fear of violence from people with mental illness
    E   There is anger among the general population towards people with mental illness

STIGMA AND CULTURE

133. Which of the following statements about locura is correct?

    A   It is an acute psychotic illness with quick resolution
    B   It is a dissociative state that follows acute trauma
    C   It is a mild, psychotic, culture-bound syndrome
    D   The condition is attributed to an inherited vulnerability
    E   It resembles the negative symptoms of schizophrenia

134. Which of the following statements is consistent with *bouffée délirante*?

    A   It has a poor prognosis
    B   It is not a classified syndrome in the ICD-10
    C   It is not a culture-bound syndrome
    D   It results in sudden and complete recovery within days
    E   It is rarely seen in black people

135. Ekbom's syndrome is a culture-bound syndrome. Which of the following statements describes it?

    A   It is a dissociative state
    B   It is found in remote eastern countries
    C   It is a monosymptomatic hypochondrical psychosis
    D   It is resistant to antipsychotics
    E   It mainly presents with a perceptual disturbance

Answers: MCQs

1. C Insensitivity to the subtleties of social intercourse

Blunting of affect refers to an inadequacy or a complete loss of all emotional life, so that patients are indifferent to their own wellbeing and that of the others. It was called 'parathymia' by Bleuler. It manifests as being socially awkward and inappropriate. Stiffening of affect refers to an initial congruent emotional response, but this does not alter as the situation changes.

2. B The symptoms must occur within 1 month of an identifiable psychosocial stressor

An adjustment disorder is a state of subjective distress and emotional disturbance, usually interfering with social functioning and performance; it arises in the period of adaptation to a significant life event or change. In children, regressive phenomena such as a return to bed-wetting, baby speech or thumb sucking are frequent presentations. Except in a prolonged depressive reaction, the symptoms do not persist for more than 6 months after cessation of the stressor and its consequences. Separation anxiety disorder of childhood is excluded from adjustment disorders.

3. C Constructional praxis

An ability to construct and organise an object from disarticulated pieces is known as constructional praxis. In the mini-mental state examination (MMSE), copying of a diagram of interlocking pentagons tests the function of constructional praxis. If the patient copies all ten angles and two pentagons intersecting, they receive a score of 1 point. Tremors and rotation are ignored in this test. Constructional apraxia is the inability to integrate and organise objects, which can occur due to right parietal lobe dysfunction.

4. A Address test

Short-term memory impairment can be assessed by tests such as the address test or the repetition of three objects. Benton's visual retention test examines the ability to copy and recall a variety of figures and shapes. Digit span, serial sevens and spelling 'world' backwards assess attention and concentration.

5. D Most patients take <2 minutes to complete their opening statement

Only 23% of patients were allowed to complete their opening statement. Most patients do not present their problems in any logical order. Most patients took <1 minute to complete their opening statement. The longer the clinician waited before interrupting the patient, the more information was elicited.

6. D Huntington's disease

In 1872, George Huntington described this eponymous disease. It is an autosomal dominant disorder that causes a combination of progressive motor, cognitive, psychiatric and behavioural dysfunction. It occurs due to an abnormality in the IT-15 gene (interesting transcript 15 gene) on chromosome A, which encodes the protein huntingtin.

7. E How have you been feeling in your spirits recently?

While conducting an interview, formal questions can be either open or closed in nature. An open question allows the patient to provide a qualitative account of his or her experience. It is commonly used to start an interview because it leads to a free flow of information which can prove to be valuable in a clinical situation.

8. A Concentration

The serial sevens test is used to assess concentration. A person is asked to take 7 away from 100 until advised to stop. The orientation test involves asking questions related to time and place.

9. B An average patient with untreated Alzheimer's disease will lose 3–4 points per year

Several patients with early dementia, on the MMSE will score well above the standard cut-off of 23 or 24 out of a total score of 30. Patients with untreated Alzheimer's dementia, on MMSE, lose on average 3–4 points. The MMSE is not a diagnostic test for dementia. It is used to measure the level of cognitive decline at the time of the examination. It is not useful to measure fronto-subcortical executive functioning. It has a significant floor and ceiling effect, so it is insufficiently discriminatory for patients with very mild or very severe cognitive impairment.

10. C Impaired consciousness

Delirium is characterised by an acute onset, fluctuating course, sleep disturbance, lability of affect, altered level of consciousness and cognitive impairment. In dementia, there is no disturbance of consciousness.

11. A Cognitive estimates test

The only test that allows a person to guess is the cognitive estimates test. In this test, a patient is asked questions such as 'What is the height of the average Irish woman?' or 'How many elephants are there in the UK?' A person has to make a guess. This is impaired in frontal lobe dysfunction, in which case patients tend to provide bizarre answers. The graded naming test, which can detect anomia, consists of line drawings in which a person is requested to name the objects in ascending difficulty. The paced auditory serial addition test assesses attention deficits. The pyramids and palm trees tests the person's semantic knowledge. The stop signal test is a test for frontal lobe executive functions. There are no guesses allowed in the above-mentioned tests apart from the cognitive estimates test.

12. C Speed of processing information

There are two components involved in reasoning, such as solving of complex problems and solving them quickly (speed). Several tests can be used to assess the speed of processing. There are two visual tests, map search and telephone search, which are used to assess mental speed. In the map search, a person has to look for target symbols on a map as fast as possible. In the telephone search, a person is asked to look for various symbols in a telephone directory as fast as possible. The paced auditory serial addition test and speed of comprehension test are other methods of assessing the speed of processing.

13. A Frontal lobes

The trail-making test is used to assess frontal lobe function. It involves asking a patient to draw a line that connects randomly placed letters or number. For example, in step one, the patient may be asked to connect A, B, C, etc. In the next stage, he will connect a-1, b-2, c-3, and so on. Performance in the trail-making test can be influenced by age, intelligence, mental speed, and attention shifting and response inhibition.

14. C Low IQ at young age is a risk factor for schizophrenia

Research studies have shown that slow IQ at a young age is a risk factor for schizophrenia. Verbal memory functioning is an important predictor of the functional outcome in schizophrenia.

Cognitive dysfunction may predate the onset of schizophrenia in many individuals. A proportion of patients with schizophrenia can have a decline in intelligence after illness. Impaired cognitive test performance in patients with schizophrenia is directly related to social deficits and it is not an epiphenomenon.

15. D Intact immediate memory

Amnestic syndrome is a group of disorders in which there is significant memory impairment compared with other cognitive functions. It is characterised by intact intelligence and intact immediate, procedural and semantic memory. In addition, there can be severe and permanent anterograde amnesia and a degree of retrograde amnesia. Persistent amnestic syndrome includes Wernicke–Korsakoff syndrome, central nervous system infections, acquired brain injury, carbon monoxide poisoning and other neurological diosorders. Transient amnestic syndrome can occur in post-traumatic stress disorder, dissociative disorder and conversion disorder. Both persistent and transient amnestic disorders can be seen after treatment with electroconvulsive therapy.

16. D Paired associative learning test

Cognitive, behavioural and memory impairement can occur in both dementia and depression. The visuospatial paired associate learning (PAL) test can accurately differentiate between dementia and depressive pseudodementia. At-risk patients for dementia who perform poorly on PAL have high rates of development of dementia. In depression, patients tend to give 'I don't know' answers to most tests.

17. E Right temporal lobe

In the clinical scenario, this patient has upper quadrantanopia. The upper visual fields, which develop from the lower retina as the image is inverted on the retina, project into the optic radiation through the temporal lobes to the lower visual cortex. A visual defect in the left upper quadrant of the visual field can occur due to a lesion in the right temporal lobe, where there is a decussation of the axons from the nasal portion of the retina at the optic chiasma.

18. E Right internuclear ophthalmoplegia

Conjugate gaze is defined as the coordinated movements of eyes bilaterally in the same direction and at the same instance. Internuclear ophthalmoplegia is an impairment in the conjugate lateral gaze wherein the eye, either left or right, fails to adduct appropriately. This results in nystagmus as the contralateral eye is able to adduct, and diplopia as the eyes diverge. It is commonly seen in multiple sclerosis. It occurs as a result of an ipsilateral lesion in the medial longitudinal fasciculus.

19. C Hyperacusis

The sensory fibres of the facial nerve, which carry taste from the anterior two-thirds of the tongue, have their cell bodies within the geniculate ganglion, situated within the facial canal of the petrous temporal bone. The motor nerve to stapedius leaves the facial nerve distal to the genu of the facial nerve. Hence, lesions within the petrous temporal bone cause the combination of loss of taste on the anterior two-thirds of the tongue and hyperacusis.

20. E Dysarthria

Pseudobulbar palsy is a term describing an upper motor neuron lesion of the lower cranial nuclei. The finding in such a patient includes:

Stiff, slow, spastic tongue (note that a fasciculation in the tongue would be consistent with a lower motor neuron lesion, as is seen in bulbar palsy)

Dysarthria (sometimes referred to as Donald Duck speech)

Emotional incontinence

Increased jaw jerk

Preserved gag and palatal reflexes.

21. E Urinary incontinence

Normal pressure hydrocephalus is a rare syndrome characterised by enlarged cerebral ventricles without cortical atrophy, dementia, urinary incontinence or gait-apraxia. It is usually seen in elderly people. The cerebrospinal fluid constituents and pressure are characteristically normal. Surgical treatment such as ventriculoperitoneal shunting occasionally helps.

22. A Electroencephalogram

The main value of an electroencephalogram (EEG) is in diagnosing epilepsy and diffuse brain disease. Spikes or spike-and-wave abnormalities are the hallmarks of epilepsy, but it should be emphasised that patients with epilepsy often have a normal EEG between seizures. An abnormal interictal EEG does not prove that one particular attack was epileptic in nature, and should not be used to make a diagnosis. Serum levels of carbamazepine and lithium will be useful in detecting the toxicity of these drugs.

23. A CT of the brain

Renal failure results in reduced excretion of nitrogenous waste products, of which urea is the most commonly measured biochemical constituent. Hyponatraemia, usually in elderly people, and possibly due to the syndrome of inappropriate secretion of antidiuretic hormone, has been associated with all types of antidepressants. However, it has been reported more frequently with selective serotonin reuptake inhibitors. From the given options, CT of the brain will help to demonstrate central tumours, intracerebral haemorrhage and infarction, subdural and extradural haematomas, cerebral atrophy, lateral shift of the middle structures, and displacements and enlargement of the ventricular system.

24. C Full blood count

Antipsychotics can potentially suppress bone marrow function and the problem is greatest with clozapine. Clozapine-induced neutropenia is reversible on discontinuation of the drug.

Agranulocytosis with clozapine is also reversible following its early detection and discontinuation of the drug, but can be fatal if allowed to persist. A full blood count will give an indication of the problem.

25. E Wechsler Adult Intelligence Scale–revised

The above-mentioned psychological instrument is used to generate verbal, performance and full scale IQs. The Wechsler adult intelligence scale–revised (WAIS-R) is used to observe the pattern of intellectual abilities that is reflected in the 11 subsets. The Minnesota multiphasic personality inventory (MMPI) generates scores on nine scales such as hypochondriasis, depression, hysteria, psychopathic deviance, masculinity/femininity, paranoia, psychasthenia (or anxiety), schizophrenia and mania. Although the MMPI was originally developed to help diagnosis, its widest use at present is more descriptive than diagnostic.

26. B Halstead–Reitan battery

The Halstead–Reitan battery is a neurological test for individuals aged 15 years and older. It consists of 13 subsets and measures a wide range of functions. The Bender visual–motor gestalt test is a projective technique consisting of nine geometrical figures that are copied by the patient. Its chief applications are to determine retardation, loss of function and organic brain deficits in children, and in the study of personality deviations that show the regressive phenomenon.

27. C Rorschach's inkblot technique

Rorschach's inkblot technique is a projective test consisting of 10 inkblots of varying designs and colours, which are shown to the patient one at a time with a request to interpret them. Its purpose is to furnish a description of the dynamic forces of personality through analysis of formal aspects of the patient's interpretations. The test yields information about the intellectual and emotional processes, the degree of personality integration and the degree to which the patient responds to environmental influences and his or her inner promptings.

28. A Childhood obesity

The main predictors of a better outcome in anorexia nervosa are a short history and onset at a younger age. Childhood obesity, low self-esteem and personality disturbances are associated with a poor outcome. A diagnosis of anorexia nervosa is probably more often missed in males. In females there is no obvious marker such as cessation of menstruation, and in males loss of sex drive occurs gradually with weight loss as testosterone falls. So-called 'reverse anorexia nervosa' or 'muscle dysmorphia' occurs almost exclusively in males.

29. A Agoraphobia

Panic attacks occur in generalised anxiety disorders, phobic anxiety disorders (most often agoraphobia), depression and acute organic disorders. Two of the DSM-IV diagnostic criteria that help to distinguish secondary anxiety attacks from panic disorder are the presence, in panic disorder, of a persistently marked concern about having further attacks and worry about the implication of the attacks. However, not all patients with agoraphobia will have panic attacks, which may be situational or spontaneous, and may meet many of the criteria for both panic disorder and agoraphobia.

30. D Between 18 and 19

Quetelet's body mass index (BMI) is calculated as:

BMI = body weight in kilograms divided by height in metres squared

In this example, BMI = 50 kg divided by (1.65 m × 1.65 m) = 18.365 kg/m^2

BMI <17.5 is one of the diagnostic features of anorexia nervosa. Recent evidence suggests that BMI has strong genetic determinants and direction of weight change in depression.

31. C Delayed insulin release

Several neuroendocrine changes are noted in a patient with anorexia nervosa. The growth hormone and the plasma cortisol levels are increased, along with a loss in normal diurnal variation. The levels of gonadotrophins are reduced. The levels of thyroxine and thyroid-stimulating hormone are usually normal, but levels of triiodothyronin (T$_3$) may be reduced. There are low levels of luteinising hormone-releasing hormone, luteinising hormone, follicle-stimulating hormone, oestrogen and progesterone.

32. A Cannabis use can precipitate schizophrenia in people who are vulnerable because of a family history of the disorder

Whether or not cannabis can predispose to later development of schizophrenia or not is a controversial issue. Some studies found that the relative risk of developing schizophrenia was 2.5 fold in users. Family history of schizophrenia may also predispose to cannabis misuse. Chronic use can lead to a state of apathy and indolence.

33. A Duration of post-traumatic amnesia

The severity of non-penetrating (closed) head injury is best assessed by the duration of post-traumatic amnesia (PTA) or anterograde amnesia, which is the interval between the injury and the return of normal day-to-day memory. It has an advantage of being reasonably accurate even when assessed retrospectively. A PTA of less than a week is associated with a reasonable outcome in most, but a PTA of more than a month often results in failure to return to work. Retrograde amnesia is less predictive of such an outcome.

34. B Four times more likely

Three major studies followed a large number of people over several years and showed that those people who use cannabis have a higher than average risk of developing schizophrenia. If a person starts smoking cannabis before the age of 15 years, there is a four times higher chance that he or she will develop a psychotic disorder before they reach 26 years of age.

35. D 2:1

Depression is common in patients who develop heart failure and is associated with a poorer prognosis if untreated. As the intensity of heart failure symptoms increases, there is an associated increase in the prevalence of depression. It is reported that 37% of older patients with congestive heart failure had major depression compared with 17% of cardiac patients without heart failure.

36. A Dorsolateral prefrontal cortex

Various brain neuroimaging studies have suggested that the negative symptoms of schizophrenia are related to hypofunction of the dorsolateral prefrontal cortex. Positron emission tomography studies indicate that there are greater metabolic abnormalities in negative symptoms compared with those noticed in positive symptoms of schizophrenia.

37. A Delirium tremens

In this clinical scenario, the retired banker has symptoms and signs suggestive of delirium tremens. It is often taken as a hallmark of alcohol dependence, but is relatively rare. It is reported to occur in about 5% of patients attending community alcohol misuse clinics. The full syndrome of delirium tremens is characterised by marked tremors of the limbs, body and tongue, restlessness, loss of contact with reality, clouding of consciousness, disorientation, and illusions that may progress to terrifying hallucinations, mostly visual but possibly auditory or tactile. The patient may experience paranoid delusions.

38. D Frontotemporal dementia

In this clinical scenario, the woman is likely to be suffering from frontotemporal dementia. This dementia is a clinically and pathologically diverse group of focal dementias presenting with the features of either frontal lobe dysfunction or temporal lobe dysfunction, or both. The patient presents with an insidious disorder of personality and behaviour, inability to focus, loss of regulation of emotions, disinhibition and utilisation behaviour. There is a relative sparing of abilities such as perception, memory (mainy immediate), praxis and spatial skills.

39. D Transient stress-related paranoid ideation

The World Health Organization's ICD-10 describes an emotionally unstable personality disorder and differentiates it into two types, such as impulsive and borderline types. It includes criteria such as chronic feelings of emptiness, involvement in intense and unstable relationships, recurrent threats or acts of self-harm, and poor self-image. Stress-related paranoia is not a criterion for this disorder in the ICD-10. In the DSM-IV, where this disorder is known as borderline personality disorder, transient stress-related paranoid ideation is included as one of the diagnostic criteria.

World Health Organization. The ICD-10 Classification of Mental and Behavioural Disorders: Clinical descriptions and diagnostic guidelines. Geneva: WHO, 1992: 198–205.

40. C High functioning autistic spectrum disorder

Individuals with Asperger's syndrome or high functioning autistic spectrum disorder (ASD) experience some speech disturbance at an earlier age. They have difficulties in social functioning and restricted discrete interests. Individuals with this disorder can be misdiagnosed as having a psychotic disorder, or schizoid or schizotypal personality disorder. Individuals usually have above-average intelligence.

41. D Hyperkinetic disorder

Individuals with a hyperkinetic disorder suffer from inattention, impulsivity and hyperactivity. There is now some loose agreement on the existence of an adult type of ADHD.

42. A Bizarre encapsulated delusions and systematised delusions

Persistent delusional disorder includes a variety of disorders in which long-standing delusions constitute the only, or the most conspicuous, clinical feature, and which cannot be classified as an organic, schizophrenic or affective disorder. Schneider's first rank symptoms or definite evidence of brain disease is incompatible with the diagnosis of persistent delusional disorder. However, the presence of occasional or transitory auditory hallucinations, particularly in elderly patients, does not rule out this diagnosis. They are also known as paranoid psychosis, paraphrenia (late-onset psychosis) and *sensitiver Beziehungswahn*.

43. E Schizophrenia and affective disorders are at the same level

According to the ICD-10 classification system, any given diagnosis excludes the presence of symptoms of higher members and includes the symptoms of lower members. There is a difference in the ICD-9 and the ICD-10 hierarchy structure, in that schizophrenia and affective disorders are placed at the same level in the ICD-10. Organic disorders are at the top and neurotic, stress-related and somatoform symptoms are at the bottom of the hierarchy.

44. D Pattern of course of schizophrenia

As there are considerable variations in the course of schizophrenia disorders, sometimes it can be coded by using a fifth character. This character can be used to specify the pattern of the course of schizophrenia. The course can be coded only after a period of observation of at least 1 year from the illness.

45. A Dissociative disorder

In the ICD-10 dissociative (conversion) disorder is coded and denoted by F 44. It includes dissociative amnesia, dissociative fugue, multiple personality disorder, dissociative (conversion) disorder not otherwise specified, dissociative stupor, trance and possession disorder, and Ganser's syndrome.

46. A Disorders of sexual preferences

The general criteria for disorders of sexual preference are:

- The individual experiences recurrent intense sexual urges and fantasies involving unusual objects or activities.
- The individual either acts on the urges or is markedly distressed by them.
- The preference has been present for at least 6 months.

47. E Schizophrenia and related disorders

In the DSM-IV, schizotypal disorder is part of the personality disorders whereas in the ICD-10 it is part of the schizophrenia spectrum disorders.

48. B Postschizophrenic depression

Disorganised schizophrenia, schizoaffective disorder and schizophreniform disorder are classified under schizophrenia and other psychotic disorders in the DSM-IV classification system.

Schizoaffective disorder is a separate category in the ICD-10 classification system. Schizoptypal disorder is a separate category in the ICD-10 and it is included under personality disorders in the DSM-IV classification system.

49. B 2 weeks

Recurrent obsessional thoughts, images or impulses or compulsive acts are the mainstay of OCD. According to the ICD-10 classification system, the symptoms should be present on most days for at least two successive weeks for a diagnosis of OCD. It should be a cause for distress and interference in regular functions. It is coded as F42 in the ICD-10 classification system.

50. C 6 months

The symptoms of generalised anxiety disorder consist of prominent tension, worry, apprehension about daily events for a period of at least 6 months, together with at least four symptoms of autonomic arousal pertaining to the chest and abdomen. It is not classified as a part of the subcategory of phobic anxiety disorders.

51. B DSM-IV only

Narcissistic personality disorder is a diagnostic category in the DSM-IV. It is not classified in the ICD-10. According to the criteria in the DSM-IV, the person has a grandiose sense of self-importance, is preoccupied with fantasies of unlimited success, believes that he is special or unique, requires excessive admiration, lacks empathy, and shows arrogant and haughty behaviour.

52. E 2 years

The features of somatisation disorder (Briquet's syndrome) are multiple, recurrent and frequently changing symptoms spread over 2 years. The symptoms emanate from multiple systems of the body. It is supported by negative investigations and several unremarkable exploratory operations might have been performed.

53. C 3 months

In delusional disorder the duration of symptoms is for a period of at least 3 months and it should not satisfy the criteria for schizophrenia. It is characterised by the development of either a single delusion or a set of related delusions, which are usually persistent and sometimes life-long. They are often persecutory, hypochondriacal, or grandiose in nature. Depressive symptoms may be present intermittently. There are transitory hallucinations which are not in the third person. Tactile and olfactory hallucinations may develop in some patients. Its onset is usually in middle age. Apart from the actions and attitudes directly related to the delusion or delusional system, affect, speech and behaviour are normal.

54. D It is relatively safe in overdose

Trazodone is rapidly absorbed (T_{max} = 1–2 hours) and prone to first-pass metabolism effects. Approximately 60–80% reaches the systemic circulation after absorption. First-pass metabolism may be saturable and the plasma levels may follow non-linear pharmacokinetics. Its major metabolite, m-chlorophenylpiperazine (mCPP), has anxiogenic properties, which counter the sedative properties of the parent compound. It is a phenylpiperazine compound with complex pharmacological actions. It blocks the reuptake of 5-HT and blocks more potently 5-HT$_{2A}$ and noradrenaline α_1- receptors. It also blocks subtypes of 5-HT$_1$ receptors. Trazodone lacks any anticholinergic activity.

55. D It is a non-competitive reversible inhibitor of acetylcholinesterase

Donepezil is well absorbed on oral ingestion and reaches a peak plasma concentration after 3–4 hours. Its half-life is approximately 72 hours. It reaches a steady–state plasma concentration after 2–3 weeks. It is highly protein bound (95%) and partly metabolised in the liver through the cytochrome P450 system. It is a highly selective for acetylcholinesterase (ACh).

56. A Clonidine withdrawal

Clonidine can lead to severe withdrawal symptoms characterised by apprehension, restlessness, abdominal pain, sweating, tremors, palpitations and headache. There may be a rapid rise in blood pressure. Usually, the symptoms start 20 hours after the last dose so it is advised that clonidine should be tapered gradually and then discontinued.

Sadock BJ, Sadock VA. Kaplan and Sadock's Synopsis of Psychiatry: Behavioral sciences/clinical psychiatry, 10th edn. Philadelphia, PA: Lippincott Williams & Wilkins, 2007: 997–1000.

57. D Noradrenaline reuptake inhibitor

Atomoxetine is a noradrenaline reuptake inhibitor. The precise mechanism of action of atomoxetine in ADHD is unknown. It exerts its pharmacological effect through the selective inhibition of the presynaptic noradrenaline transporter, therefore inhibiting the reuptake of noradrenaline. Stimulant medication approved for ADHD in children and adults works through increasing systemic levels of dopamine by binding to dopamine receptors in the brain.

58. E Trazodone

Trazadone and alprazolam are triazolopyridines drugs. Amoxapine is a tetracyclic drug. Dothiepin and amitriptyline are tricyclic drugs. Diazepam is a benzodiazepine drug.

59. A Amitriptyline

Imipramine, amitriptyline, trimipramine, clomipramine and doxapine are tertiary amines. Amoxapine, desipramine, nortriptyline and protripyline are secondary amines.

60. B α_1-Receptor blockade

Priapism is a painful erection of the penis that persists in the absence of physical and psychological stimulation. Blockade of α_1-receptors leads to dysregulation of smooth muscle tone in the penile vascular tissue. This can cause venous outflow obstruction in corpora cavernosa and thus priapism. Priapism can be caused by antipsychotic medications such as clozapine and chlorpromazine, and antidepressant medications such as trazodone, antihypertensive medications, anticoagulants and drugs such as cocaine, alcohol and opiates.

61. E Sigma receptors

Fluvoxamine is an antidepressant medication that acts as a selective serotonin reuptake inhibitor. Sigma-1 and sigma-2 receptors are a separate group of receptors. Fluvoxamine acts as a sigma-1-receptor agonist in the brain. This helps to improve cognition and depression symptoms.

62. C Exceeding the rate of recommended dose escalation

Lamotrigine-induced rash can occur in 5–10% of patients. It usually presents as a maculopapular or morbilliform rash and can lead to serious life-threatening consequences. It usually occurs 2–6 weeks after treatment. The risk factors for lamotrigine-induced rash are young age, combining lamotrigine with valproic acid, exceeding the recommended starting dose and exceeding the rate of recommended dose escalation. Lamotrigine-induced rash usually resolves on withdrawal of the treatment with lamotrigine.

63. D Topiramate

Renal stones, mainly calcium phosphate stones, can occur following treatment with topiramate. It has been used as a mood stabiliser in treatment of bipolar affective disorder, in addition to epilepsy and migraine. It acts as a carbonic anhydrase inhibitor and can cause metabolic acidosis, decrease citrate excretion and increase urinary pH. This can give rise to renal stones.

64. E Vigabatrin

This is a γ-aminobutyric acid transaminase inhibitor. It can cause retinal cone system dysfunction, which can lead to constriction of peripheral field of vision and blurring as side effects. These symptoms may be irreversible and persistent.

65. E Tachycardia

Patients who misuse heroin can develop withdrawal symptoms due to concurrent use of buprenorphine. This phenomemon is known as 'precipitated withdrawal'. All the symptoms mentioned in the question are of opioid intoxication symptoms except tachycardia, which is an opioid withdrawal symptom.

66. D 6–9 months of age

During the later part of first year after birth, the infant shows specific attachment towards the primary caregiver and which is usually the mother. The infant starts orienting to his or her mother at the age of 2–3 months and allows strangers to handle them when one or more people are present. Many of the studies showed that children develop specific attachment from the age of 6–9 months. After the age of 3 years, attachment behaviour starts declining and is less prominent.

67. E Secure

Ainsworth conducted the strange situation experiment with two separations and two reunion episodes. According to the infant's behaviour, it is classified as type A, B or C. Type A is an avoidant type of attachment, where the child is highly oriented towards the environment. Type B is a secure attachment, where the child plays independently when the mother is in the vicinity, may get distressed when she leaves and seeks contact on her return. Type C is a resistant or ambivalent type of attachment, where the child is highly mother/caregiver directed and displays low playful behaviour.

68. B Dismissing

Main's Adult Attachment Interview predicts the infantile attachment pattern using analysis of adults' recollection of their childhoods. The secure attachment is also called autonomous attachment. Adults who had a secure attachment were able to talk freely, provided spontaneous, coherent answers and had a non-defensive approach. Adults, who had a dismissing type of attachment often minimised their experience, were not able to elaborate and were found to be giving 'I don't know' type-answers. Adults who had a preoccupied type of attachment, had insecure and ambivalent attachment. Their responses were emotionally dominated, with lengthy discussions of childhood memories. Adults who had a disorganised type of attachment had broken and interrupted logical flow of thoughts. They became irrational or incoherent.

69. D Preoccupied

Secure attachment is also called autonomous attachment. People who had secure attachment were able to talk freely and provided spontaneous and coherent answers, and were non-defensive.

Dismissing: they often minimise their experience, were not able to elaborate and were found to be giving 'I don't know'-type answers.

Preoccupied: they had insecure and ambivalent attachment. Their responses were emotionally dominated with lengthy discussions of childhood memories.

Disorganised: broken and interrupted logical flow of thoughts was seen in these people. People became irrational or incoherent.

70. E Slow to warm up

According to the Chess study, three types of behavioural styles can be explained by observing childhood temperaments. These are as follows:

1. **Easy temperament:** this is characterised by the regular rhythmic pattern of needs where a child adopts well, is active and shows a low intensity of emotions.
2. **Difficult temperament:** this is characterised by a child presenting with an irregular biorhythm, negative mood and being uncomfortable with new experiences.
3. **Slow to warm up temperament:** this is characterised by a child who adapts poorly to change, and has slow changes in mood, somewhat regular habits and mild intensity of emotions.

71. D Short-term memory uses visual coding

Short-term memory largely uses acoustic coding. All other options mentioned in the question are correct in relation to short-term memory. Furthermore, loss of information from short-term memory occurs due to displacement and decay.

72. A Episodic memory

This form of memory represents an autobiographical memory; it depends on people's personal and global events of life. Procedural memory is also known as an implicit memory. It is made up of skills and habits such as riding a bicycle or swimming. Semantic memory is the factual knowledge of the world, e.g. when did the First World War take place.

73. E It has a short capacity

Sensory memory has a large capacity but it can be disrupted by inflow of new information into the same modality. All the other options mentioned in the question are true for sensory memory.

74. D Reduction

Retrieval is described as the period when the information is brought into the short-term memory from the long-term memory. It contains recognition, which is similar to solving MCQs. Recall is described as actively searching and reproducing the information. Reintegration or reconstruction is the recollection of the experiences based on certain cues.

75. B Formal operational stage

Table 2.1 Summary of Piaget's stages of cognitive development

Stage	Age	Important tasks	Experiment
Sensorimotor	Birth to 2 years	Circular reactions Development of object permanence Beginning of symbolic thought	Hiding objects
Preoperational	2–7 years	1. Egocentrism 2. Centration 3. Irreversibility	1. Mountain task 2. Conservation task
Concrete operational	7–11 years	Attains most conservation operations Unable to use abstract concepts	Classification of objects according to rules (seriation)
Formal operational	11+ years	Capable of abstract thought, e.g. deductive reasoning, hypothesis testing	Pendulum experiment

76. E Object permanence is completed at 18 months

Egocentrism refers to the tendency to view the world from one's own perspective and the inability to understand the world from other people's points of view. Castration anxiety is associated with the phallic stage of Freud's psychosexual development stages, which develops between the ages of 3 and 5 years. Abstract reasoning, logical thinking and hypothesis testing are seen in the formal operational stage. Conservation of volume, number, length and mass is associated with the concrete operational stage.

77. C Stage 4

Kohlberg's has described six stages of moral development. These are as follows:

1. Obedience and punishment orientation
2. Individualism and exchange (reward orientation)
3. Concordance orientation (good boy/good girl orientation)
4. Maintaining social order and law
5. Social laws and individual rights
6. Universal principles of justice

78. C Temperament

Thomas and Chess conceptualised temperament as representing the behavioural style in children–'the show of behaviour'. In the 30-year-long New York Longitudinal Study of Observing, nine categories of dimensions (e.g. activity level, adaptability, mood and others) categorised temperament into three types:

- Easy temperament 40%
- Difficult temperament 10%

- Slow to warm up 15% and
- Rest ungrouped 35%

The concept of attachment was described by John Bowlby. The concept of object constancy is associated with Margaret Mahler. Imprinting was described by Lorenz.

79. B Long-term memory is also known as secondary or remote memory

Memory is divided into short-term and long-term memory. Long-term memory is also known as recent past memory, secondary memory, remote memory and recent memory. Working memory is also known as short-term memory. The capacity for short-term memory is 5–9 bits. Short- and long-term memory differs for information that they store, with the capacity for short-term memory being limited.

80. D It implies incongruity in a person's beliefs, knowledge and behaviour

Cognitive dissonance produces an uncomfortable tension state and is concerned with a person changing his or her thinking to reduce disharmony. Attribution theory is a cognitive approach concerned with how people perceive the causes of behaviour. In this, the person is likely to attribute others' behaviour to situational causes.

81. B It is a paradigm used to explain psychosis in depressed individuals

The concept of learned helplessness was first described by Martin Seligman. It is a paradigm that is used to explain depression in individuals who feel helpless, with no options, and are unable to control events. It teaches an individual that there is no way to avoid an aversive stimulus.

82. A Authority

French and Raven have described five types of social power:

1. **Authority/legitimate:** this is the power derived from the role or positional power. Managers, doctors and prime ministers all have legitimate power that comes with their roles.
2. **Reward:** this is the power derived from the ability to allocate resources. Your employer or educational supervisor can reward you in different ways.
3. **Coercive:** this is the power to punish. This form forces an individual to do something against his or her will. Think dictator, bully or parent! (It is not necessarily negative.)
4. **Referent:** this power is derived from another person liking you or wanting to be like you, e.g. celebrities and local social leaders. It is being charismatic and liked by others.
5. **Expert:** this power is derived from skills, knowledge and experience. A trade union could enforce this kind of power if they encouraged their members to strike for better conditions.

83. D Referent

French and Raven have described the following five types of social powers:

1. **Authority/Legitimate:** power derived from role (as above). Managers, doctors and prime ministers all have legitimate power that comes with their roles.
2. **Reward:** power derived from the ability to allocate resources. Your employer or educational supervisor can reward you in different ways.

3. **Coercive:** power to punish. This is the power that forces someone to do something against his or her will. Think dictator, bully or parent! (It is not necessarily negative.)
4. **Referent:** charismatic and liked by others. This power is derived from another person liking you or wanting to be like you, e.g. celebrities and local social leaders.
5. **Expert:** power derives from skill, knowledge and experience. This power comes from having the knowledge and skills that someone else requires. A trade union could enforce this kind of power if they encouraged their members to strike for better conditions.

84. E Self-image

Argyle (1994) has explained the four dimension of self. Self-image is what the self supposes itself to be. It may differ from real self and it is related to factors such as gender, identity and the role played by the individuals. Self-esteem is the value that one attaches to oneself. Ego-self is what one would ideally like to be. Integration of self is the consistency of the various dimensions of the self. Self-concept is one's full descriptive concept of oneself.

85. C Thurstone's scale

This scale consists of statements that have been ranked and assigned values. Patients select one with which they agree the most and a mean score is derived. The scale is associated with bias in ranking. Likert's scale is a five-point scale. The semantic differential scale consists of nine or more paired bipolar adjectives and, for each, there is a five-point visual analogue scale, on which patients mark their response. In sociometry, patients in a group nominate preferred partners and create sociograms, which identify subgroups.

86. C Premorbid intelligence

The national adult reading test, The Cambridge contextual reading test, the spot the word test and the Wechsler test of adult reading are used to test premorbid IQ. These tests are based on the observations that reading ability is relatively preserved and resistant to the effects of brain damage. They may give some indication of premorbid attainment levels.

87. D PSE provides an operational definition of symptoms to be rated

Present state examination (PSE) is a semi-structured interview, which probes for each symptom and has a detailed list of signs to be evaluated. These signs are generally rated as absent, mild/possible and moderate/definite. It covers only the past 4 weeks, unless augmented by additional duration questions. There is a computer program, known as 'CATEGO', which can generate diagnoses for the major disorders except personality disorders, in children, adolescents and individuals with a learning disability. Schedule for affective disorders and schizophrenia (SADS) is a structured rating scale with symptom-rating criteria contained within the interview schedule. The symptom severity is assessed on a seven-point scale where three or more is usually 'clinically significant' for the current episode, previous week, point of maximal severity and previous episode. SADS is not useful for organic disorders or anorexia nervosa.

88. D Present state examination

The PSE is a semi-structured interview providing an objective assessment of patients' symptoms. Beck's depression inventory is a self-rating scale, invented by Aaron Beck for assessment of the severity of depression. Leyton's obsessional inventory is a self-rated questionnaire for assessment of obsessional symptoms. The severity of alcohol dependence questionnaire is a self-administered rating scale designed by the World Health Organization for measuring the severity of alcohol dependence. The general health questionnaire is suitable for screening for psychiatric morbidity in the general population. Initially, potential cases are identified using a self-rated questionnaire. Once caseness is suspected, detailed interviews or other diagnostic tools are used to confirm a diagnosis.

89. D Functional analysis of behaviour is an absolute necessity

Functional analysis consists of a highly detailed account of current determinants of the problem. It aims to define the problem and identify the key variables. It uses a subjective account of the antecedents of problems perceived by the patient. It uses the assumption that immediate consequences are the key determinants of behaviour.

90. A A smooth pattern of behaviour is found with a variable–ratio schedule

The term 'schedule of reinforcement' refers to the fact that in many situations not every response is reinforced. In a fixed-interval schedule, individuals are typically rewarded with money for their work, say once a week or month. In a fixed-ratio schedule people are rewarded on the piecework that they produce.

91. B It is an activity adopted by those who consider themselves to be ill

Society bestows a special role on people who are ill. Parsons (1951) termed this concept 'sick role', which is made up of two privileges and two duties, as follows:

- Exemption from certain social responsibilities
- The right to expect help and care from others
- The obligation to seek help and care from others
- The expectation of a desire to recover.

When the person is ill, the sick role is adaptive. However, if the person continues in the sick role after the illness is over, recovery is delayed as the individual continues to avoid responsibilities and depends on others, instead of becoming independent.

92. D Patient's interpretation of life events is responsible for anxiety

Cognitive theory proposes that generalised anxiety disorder arises from a tendency to worry excessively and unproductively about problems, and to focus on potentially threatening circumstances. Three kinds of cognitions are considered in the treatment.

- **Fear of fear:** general concerns about the effects of being anxious, e.g. losing control.
- **Fear of symptoms:** concerns about specific symptoms, e.g. fear that palpitations are a sign of heart disease.
- **Fear of negative evaluation:** concerns that other people will react unfavourably.

93. C Hormone replacement therapy

Various environmental factors are associated with an altered risk for developing Alzheimer's disease. However, for many of them, it is not clear to what extent they are causal, act independently or interact with a genetic predisposition. The negative associations with an exposure to non-steroidal anti-inflammatory drugs and hormone replacement therapy (HRT) are quite strong. The inverse association with HRT may be confounded by the fact that HRT users are more likely to be well educated and healthy. Low educational attainment, a history of head injury, cerebrovascular disease, depression or diabetes mellitus, and high homocysteine levels are risk factors for dementia.

94. C Prolonged education

Poor education in men has been shown to increase the risk of Alzheimer's disease (AD).

It is thought that poorer linguistic ability in those who developed AD was in fact a very early manifestation of the disease. Superior premorbid intellect and education may protect against AD. The *APoEε2* allele is possibly protective against AD, although the evidence is not conclusive. Physical activity may also be protective against AD. Patients with Down's syndrome develop AD before the age of 40 years, although a cognitive decline is often not seen until a later age.

95. C Higher number of previous depressive episodes

The best predictor of the future course of depression is the history of previous episodes. Not surprisingly, the risk of recurrence is much greater in those with several previous episodes. Other factors include:

- Incomplete symptomatic resolution
- Bipolar affective disorder
- Early age of onset
- Poor social support
- Poor physical health
- Comorbid substance misuse
- Comorbid personality disorder.

96. C Preventive measures targeted at high-risk individuals produces the best pay-off for those individuals, but the best pay-off for the population as a whole is provided by universal measures

Alcohol problems are endemic in most industrialised nations. The efficacy of treatment for alcohol problems is uncertain so prevention should be better than a cure. Prevention is most visibly effective when a specific effect can be traced to a cause that is readily amenable to influence or treatment. Focusing a preventive strategy only on those at 'high risk' would have less impact on the overall level of harm than a population-based approach. This is termed the 'preventive paradox'.

97. B Automatic obedience

In automatic obedience, patients carry out all the instructions regardless of the consequences. A stereotyped movement is a repetitive, non-goal-directed action that is carried out in a uniform way. A mannerism is the unusual repeated performance of a goal-directed motor action, or the maintenance of an unusual modification of an adaptive posture. In echopraxia, the patient imitates the interviewer's every action, despite the interviewer asking him or her not to do so. In advertence, the patient turns towards the interviewer when she or he addresses the patient.

98. C Recognition

This phenomenon refers to the retrieval of stored information from memory which depends on the identification of items previously learned. Déjà-vu is a feeling of familiarity in an unfamiliar situation. Jamais-vu is the opposite of déjà-vu—there is unfamiliarity with a familiar place.

Jamais-vu can occur as a normal experience or in conditions such as temporal lobe epilepsy, and cerebrovascular and neurotic disorders, which are not primarily memory disorders. Registration is the capacity to add new information to the memory store. Retention is the ability to maintain knowledge that can be subsequently returned to consciousness.

99. A Delusion of control

Delusional disorder is characterised by the presence of a delusion or a set of related delusions other than those listed for the typical schizophrena diagnosis under F20 in the ICD-10 (i.e. other than completely impossible or culturally inappropriate). Delusion of control is a typical schizophrenia delusion under the F20 category of the ICD-10. Therefore it suggests a diagnosis of schizophrenia rather than a delusional disorder. Other delusions mentioned in the question are not described as typical of schizophrenia, and so can be part of a delusional disorder.

100. B Clock drawing

The MMSE does not include the clock-drawing test. This test is a useful cognitive test for parietal lobe functioning. Working memory includes temporary storage and manipulation of visual and spatial information, and holding memory traces of verbal information for a couple of seconds, combined with subvocal rehearsal. In MMSE, working memory and concentration are assessed by the serial sevens test. Reading and writing have separate tasks in the MMSE. Apraxia is tested by asking the patient to copy two intersecting pentagons.

101. A Cotard's syndrome

In this clinical scenario, the woman has symptoms that suggest Cotard's syndrome. This syndrome is the association of hypochondriacal and nihilistic delusions with depressive psychosis in elderly people. It is not one of the first rank symptoms, but may take the form of a tactile hallucination, a delusion or an overvalued idea. It is not a primary delusion because it appears in the context of depressed mood. In Ekbom's syndrome, the patient believes that he or she is infested with small but macroscopic organisms. Couvade's syndrome is an abnormality of the experience of self in which a male spouse/partner complains of obstetric symptoms during his partner's pregnancy and parturition. It is not a delusion.

102. C An obsession with dirt or germs, followed by washing or avoidance

Obsessions are recurrent, intrusive, and distressing thoughts, images or impulses, whereas compulsions are repetitive, seemingly purposeful behaviours that a person feels driven to perform. Obsessions are usually unpleasant and increase a person's anxiety, whereas carrying out compulsions reduces anxiety. Resistance to carrying out a compulsion results in increased anxiety. The patient usually realises that the obsessions are irrational and experiences both the obsession and the compulsion as egodystonic. The most common pattern is an obsession with dirt or germs, followed by washing or avoiding presumably contaminated objects (door knobs, electrical switches, newspapers, people's hands, telephones). The feared object is hard to avoid (e.g. faeces, urine, dust or germs). Patients wash their hands excessively and sometimes avoid leaving home because of their fear of germs.

103. E *Vorbeireden*

This was first described by Ganser. In the choice of answers, the patient appears deliberately to pass over the indicated correct answer and selects a false one, which any child could recognise as such. It is a rare phenomenon and more likely to be seen in those awaiting trial. Verbigeration is repetition of words or syllables that expressive aphasic patients may use while desperately searching for the correct word. Dementia is characterised by a progressive decline in intellectual functions. Cryptamnesia is the experience of not remembering that one is remembering. Confabulation is the falsification of memory occurring in clear consciousness in association with an organically derived amnesia.

104. A Decoding

Encoding or registration is the capacity to add new information to the memory store. Storage or retention is the ability to maintain knowledge that can subsequently be returned to consciousness. Retrieval is the capacity to access stored information from the memory by recognition or recall. Rehearsal is a term used to refer to mental techniques for helping to remember information, e.g. continuously repeating the material to be remembered. Decoding is not described as one of the steps in memorising things.

105. A Mannerisms

These are unusual repeated performances of a goal-directed motor action or the maintenance of an unusual modification of an adaptive posture. The action, in question, is similar to saluting, which is a goal-directed movement. A stereotyped movement is a repetitive, non-goal-directed action that is carried out in a uniform way. Tardive dyskinesia is a side effect of long-term treatment with antipsychotics, usually characterised by repetitive purposeless movements of the muscles of the face, mouth and tongue. Tics are rapid, repetitive, coordinated and stereotyped movements. In *mitmachen*, the body can be put into any position without any resistance on the part of the patient, although they may have been instructed to resist all movements.

106. D Perception

Déjà vu is a feeling of familiarity in an unfamiliar situation. Jamais vu is opposite of déjà vu. These can occur as normal experiences or in temporal lobe epilepsy, cerebrovascular disorders and neurotic disorders. These are not primarily memory disorders. These are similar to sensory distortion of derealisation. The situation is perceived as if familiar or new. Therefore, this involves perception. This experience is not related to volition, behaviour or cognition. Even though they are associated with affective changes, they are not primarily mood disorders.

107. B Thought broadcasting

This is thought broadcasting because the woman believes that her thoughts leave her mind and diffuse widely so that other people receive them. Thought insertion is the belief that thoughts are being placed in the mind from outside. Thought withdrawal is the belief that thoughts are being taken away from the person against his or her will. Thought echo is a form of hallucination in which one's own thoughts are audible.

108. D Voices asking the patient to go to London and meet the Queen

This is an example of a command hallucination, which is not classified as a first rank symptom. It may be seen in conditions such as schizophrenia and severe depression. *Écho de la pensée* is the French term used for thought echo. Delusional perception and somatic passivity are also first rank symptoms.

109. C Haptic hallucination

This is an example of an unpleasant from of haptic (touch) hallucination, also known as formication. This form of hallucination is most commonly associated with drug-induced states, or withdrawal symptoms from alcohol and cocaine. It is often associated with delusion of infestation. Delirium tremens is an alcoholic withdrawal syndrome characterised by gross changes in perception, mood and the conscious states. Lilliput's hallucinations are hallucinations of little animals or diminutive men, but are usually associated with amusement and delight. Kinaesthetic hallucination involves a sense of joints or muscles.

110. A Affect illusion

This is an example of an affect illusion, which arises in the context of a particular mood state such as anxiety. Completion illusion depends on inattention such as misreading words because one would read the word as if it were complete. Pareidolic illusion is a vivid illusion without any effort. Pseudoillusion is just a distractor in the question.

111. A Capgras' syndrome

This is an example of Capgras' syndrome. The person believes that another person, usually closely related to him or her, has been replaced by an exact double, an imposter who looks exactly the same. Fregoli's syndrome is the delusional misidentification of an unfamiliar person as a familiar one, even though there is no physical resemblance. The syndrome of intermetamorphosis is the delusional belief that others undergo radical changes in physical and psychological identity, culminating in a different person altogether. The syndrome of subjective doubles is the delusional belief in the existence of physical duplicates of the self.

112. B Ineffective decoding

Ineffective registration or encoding could be due to lack of attention, so information is not learned in the first place. Decay refers to the fading of memory traces with time. The Interference theory of forgetting proposes that people forget because of competition from other material learned previously or subsequently. The tendency to forget things, i.e. one does not want to remember, is motivated by forgetting which is similar to repression in freudian terms. Decoding is not described in memory or forgetting.

113. B Concrete thinking

This is an example of impaired abstraction leading to concrete thinking. The patient explains sideways walking as caused by side effects, thus failing to understand the actual meaning of side effects but taking them literally. The loss of ego boundaries is related to delusions and hallucinations and can be seen in schizophrenia. Insight and judgement are not related to this behaviour.

114. B Projection

This is the defence against unpalatable anxieties, impulses or attributes in one's own psyche, which are attributed to an external origin. The internal threats are externalised and are then easier to manage. Narcissism is the absorption with self and excessive self-love, which arises in the presence of feelings of insecurity about the self. The concentration of interest on self and administration of the person impairs other interpersonal relationships.

115. E Social anxiety disorder

In conversion disorder, the conversion of emotional distress into physical symptoms with a symbolic meaning is considered to be one of the aetiological factors. Freud suggested that loss of an 'object', some abstraction or internal representation, is associated with depression. He proposed that obsessional symptoms occur when there is regression to the anal stage of development, as a way of avoiding impulses related to the subsequent genital and oedipal stages. Anxiety is reduced by the action of repression and reaction formation.

116. E Unconscious

All psychic material not in the immediate field of awareness is in the unconscious. The unconscious is the reservoir of psychic representatives of the drives and all phylogenic acquisitions. It operates on the pleasure principle and primary process thinking. Ego is the mediator between the person and reality, and adaptation to it. It is the executive organ of the reality principle and is ruled by secondary process thinking. Ego-ideal is the part of the super-ego that includes the rules and standards for good behaviours, e.g. parental discipline. Super-ego is the representative of society within the psyche and includes ideal aspirations (ego-ideal). It is mainly unconscious and its functions include: approval or disapproval of the ego's actions; critical self-observation; demands that the ego repent or make reparation for wrong doing; and self-love or self-esteem as the ego reward for having done right.

117. D Projection

This involves attributing unwanted ideas or feelings that are experienced within oneself to others. Archetypically, this involves attributing to others the negative emotions that one has towards them. Projection is often seen as a mechanism by which patients refuse to accept responsibility for their own mistakes and instead place the blame on others.

118. B It is commonly used by the child to manage anxiety

Winnicott conceived the idea of transitional phenomena occurring in a potential space located between the boundaries of self (inner world) and the boundaries of an object (external world). It is an early indication of the capacity to see the self as separate from the object, and to manipulate external objects and events. The transitional object comes into use when the child is aged between 4 and 18 months. It symbolises the interplay of separateness and unity.

119. C Kahlbaum

In catatonia, peculiarities of movements are the characteristic feature–usually rigidity. Waxy flexibility, mannerism, negativism and posturing are a few of the catatonic symptoms seen in patients with schizophrenia and severe depression. Kahlbaum coined the term 'catatonia.' Dementia praecox is the term coined by Kraepelin. Bleuler coined the term 'schizophrenia'. Hecker coined the term 'hebephrenic schizophrenia'.

120. C Deniker

Chorpromazine is from the thiorazine group. It was introduced by Delay and Deniker in the mid-1950s. This was the first drug that significantly reduced the symptoms of psychosis. Kane is associated with clozapine and John Cade with the discovery of lithium for the treatment of mental illnesses.

121. D Kurt Schneider

He proposed and described the first rank symptoms of schizophrenia. These are neither diagnostic nor prognostic, but are indicative of schizophrenia. The first rank symptoms are thought insertion, thought withdrawal, thought broadcasting, delusion of perception, passivity phenomena, third person auditory hallucinations and running commentary. The term 'schizophrenia' was coined by Eugene Bleuler in 1911. Carl Schneider described different forms of formal thought disorders.

122. C Hecker

Hebephrenic schizophrenia is a type of schizophrenia in which affective changes are prominent. The mood is shallow and inappropriate, and thoughts are disorganised. The onset is usually in adolescence. Hecker described hebephrenic schizophrenia. Bleuler coined the term 'schizophrenia'. Griesinger developed views about the neuropathological basis of mental disorders. William Tuke promoted moral treatment for psychiatric patients.

123. D Ribot

Anhedonia is a lack of pleasure in doing activities that were previously enjoyable. Ribot coined the term 'anhedonia'. Sifneos coined the term 'alexithymia', which is difficulty in verbalising emotions. Moreno is considered to be a father of psychodrama. Kahlbaum described cyclothymia, which is persistent instability of mood involving periods of depression and mild elation, but none of them is severe or prolonged enough to fulfil the diagnosis of bipolar affective disorder.

124. A Carl Schneider

Kurt Schneider proposed first rank symptoms of schizophrenia. These are neither diagnostic nor prognostic but are indicative of schizophrenia .The first rank symptoms are thought insertion, thought withdrawal, thought broadcasting, delusion of perception, passivity phenomena, third person auditory hallucinations and running commentary. Eugene Bleuler coined the term 'schizophrenia' in 1911. Carl Schneider described different forms of formal thought disorder.

125. C 1943

Maslow mainly concentrated on a person's experience of the world. He postulated Maslow's triangle, which is represented by the hierarchy of needs, in which, to reach the higher level, the lower level must be satisfied. This important theory was put forward in the year 1943.

126. D Modecate (fluphenazine decanoate)

The first depot antipsychotic, Modecate was introduced in 1967. Haloperidol depot injection is also among the first few depot injections. The other recent, typical, depot antipsychotic injections are flupenthixol and zuclopentixol. Risperidal Consta (risperidone) is an atypical depot injection.

127. A Bradford Hill

Bradford Hill discovered the experimental design called the randomised controlled trial (RCT). It is the most important tool in today's evidence-based medicine, which is gaining momentum particularly in psychiatry. John Cade discovered the antimanic effects of lithium in 1948, which he observed while injecting the guinea-pigs with the urine of patients with mania when he noticed the calming effects of lithium (as its uric acid salt). Leonard, in 1957, divided mood disorder into 'unipolar' and 'bipolar' forms. Delay and Deniker, in 1952, reported the effects of chlorpromazine in psychosis. Paul Janssen (1958), a Belgian clinician and chemist, synthesised and introduced haloperidol as an antipsychotic.

128. C Imipramine

This was used as the first antidepressant in 1958 by Robert Kuhn. Iproniazid was the first monoamine inhibitor (MAOI) to be used in 1957 and was called a 'psychic energiser'. The Swiss drug manufacturer Geigy Pharmaceuticals, now called Novartis, developed clomipramine from imipramine in the 1960s.

129. D Kasanin

Jacob Kasanin introduced the term 'schizoaffective disorder' in 1933 to refer to a disorder with symptoms of both schizophrenia and mood disorders. The onset was often sudden and occurred early in life. Kasanin observed that these patients had a good premorbid level of functioning and often a specific stressor preceded its onset.

130. B Cade

In 1949, John FJ Cade noticed that lithium urate caused lethargy in animals. Later, he carried out research on the successful therapeutic effects on patients with manic episodes. Mogen Schou demonstrated, in the 1950s and 1960s, the short-term prophylactic effect of lithium for bipolar disorder.

131. C Need to hide the condition from others

It is actually women who suffer more stigma of mental illness in the Indian subcontinent. A family history of mental illness can be a major factor for stigma. There is a fear of rejection by neighbours. Stigma is related to the fear of marital prospects. Young people are more stigmatised than older people.

132. D There is a fear of violence about people with mental illness

There are limited studies examining the prejudice against people with mental illness. The evidence highlights the public fear of violence among this population. The rest of the options are not correct because there is very little evidence to support it.

133. D The condition is attributed to an inherited vulnerability

This is a severe and chronic psychosis with an inherited vulnerability. It usually occurs in response to ongoing multiple life difficulties. The patient exhibits perceptual disturbances such as auditory and visual hallucinations. The patient may be agitated, incoherent, violent and unpredictable, and unable to follow rules of social interaction.

134. A It has a poor prognosis

Bouffée délirante is an acute and transient psychotic reaction that occurs in response to a stressful event. It is usually seen in West Africa and Haiti. It commonly presents as psychomotor agitation. The patient may become acutely muddled and confused with episodic aggression. The presentation may be accompanied by visual and auditory hallucinations or paranoid ideation.

135. C It is a monosymptomatic hypochondrical psychosis

Ekbom's syndrome is a psychotic state when a person starts believing that he or she is infested with parasites (delusional parasitosis). It was described by JP Webb Jr in 1993. The patient may present with perceptual disturbances of parasites crawling inside the skin, as seen in formication. It usually occurs in elderly women. Treatment is with antipsychotic agents, psychotherapy and working together with a dermatologist.

Chapter 3

Test questions: 3

Questions: MCQs

For each question, select one answer option.

HISTORY AND MENTAL STATE EXAMINATION

1. During an assessment interview, the clinician asked a 23-year-old man questions such as, 'What did your mother say when your father said this to your brother?'. Which interview technique is used in this case?

    A   Closed question
    B   Circular question
    C   Direct question
    D   Open question
    E   Put-down question

2. During a therapy session of a family consisting of the couple, two daughters and a son, the son had been quiet and said very little, if anything. On the other hand, the couple and their daughters tended to fill the silence by saying almost anything, or having a silly laugh. The therapist then asked the couple, 'If your son spoke now what might he say?'. Which interview technique is used in this case?

    A   Facilitation
    B   Hypothetical question
    C   Interpretation
    D   Positive reinforcement
    E   'Run-on' questioning

3. A 21-year-old man told his doctor that Jesus spoke to him whenever he started his motorbike and stopped talking to him whenever he switched the engine off. He found this very distressing and confusing, so could not use his motorbike to go to work. Which of the following explains this experience?

    A   Affective illusion
    B   Anxious foreboding
    C   Extracampine hallucination
    D   Functional hallucination
    E   Kinaesthetic hallucination

4. A 37-year-old single American man informed his doctor that, whenever he saw President Obama on television, he got sharp pains in his right leg. He was convinced that President Obama was controlling him through the television. Which of the following can explain this man's experience?

    A   Hemisomatognosis
    B   Hyperschemazia

    C   Hyposchemazia
    D   Paraschemazia
    E   Reflex hallucination

5.   A 61-year-old business executive had an exploratory laparotomy 5 days ago. He told the nurses that he saw tiny pink elephants and white tigers dancing outside the windowsills. He has a history of alcohol dependence. Which of the following explains his experience?

    A   Hypnagogic hallucinations
    B   Hypnopompic hallucinations
    C   Lilliputian hallucinations
    D   Paraschemazia
    E   Pareidolia

6.   Which of the following is an example of a closed question?

    A   'Have you been sleeping well?'
    B   'How are your sleep and appetite?'
    C   'So, do I understand this correctly that … ?'
    D   'What brought you to the emergency department today?'
    E   'You were not sleeping at that time?'

7.   What does the three-stage command in the mini-mental state examination (MMSE) test?

    A   Concentration
    B   Delayed recall
    C   Language naming
    D   Language understanding
    E   Verbal fluency

8.   A 48-year-old married man was concerned that he might be developing Parkinson's disease. Which of the following clinical features is diagnostic?

    A   A 10- to 12-Hz resting tremor
    B   Board-like muscular rigidity
    C   Exaggerated arm swinging
    D   Facial hypomimia
    E   Macrographia

9.   Which of the following is the most appropriate and quickest assessment test for performance IQ?

    A   MMSE
    B   National adult reading test
    C   Raven's progressive matrices
    D   Stanford–Binet scale
    E   Wechsler adult intelligence scale IV

10. Which of the following statements about Addenbrooke's cognitive examination is correct?

    A   Possible outcomes include delirium, dementia and depression with psychotic symptoms
    B   Scores of < 82 predict dementia with 100% specificity
    C   Scores of < 82 predict dementia with 100% sensitivity
    D   Scores of < 90 predict dementia with 100% sensitivity
    E   The MMSE should be conducted separately

11. Which of the following is assessed by the clock-drawing test?

    A   Attention
    B   Comprehension

C   Concentration
D   Insight
E   Orientation to time and person

12. You are assessing the language function in a 50-year-old man with a history of cerebrovascular accident. He says 'litter for letter'. What is this an example of?

A   Nominal aphasia
B   Phonemic paraphasia
C   Semantic deficit
D   Semantic paraphasia
E   Superordinate response

13. Which of the following is a non-verbal test for semantic memory?

A   Boston naming test
B   Cactus and camel test
C   Category fluency test
D   Similarities test
E   Word-to-picture matching

14. Which of the following can be assessed by the word stem completion task?

A   Declarative memory
B   Episodic memory
C   Priming
D   Semantic memory
E   Working memory

15. Which of the following lobe functions is assessed by the Iowa gambling test assess?

A   Frontal lobe
B   Left parietal lobe
C   Left temporal lobe
D   Right parietal lobe
E   Right temporal lobe

16. A 31-year-old man presented with a spinal injury. On examination, you diagnosed that he had spastic paralysis of the lower limbs. You tested his sensations and found that he had sensation above the umbilicus. Where is the spinal cord lesion?

A   C4
B   L3
C   S1
D   T4
E   T10

17. Which of the following is present in the Brown–Séquard syndrome with a right-sided lesion?

A   Decreased reflexes on the right
B   Left hemiplegia of the arm and leg
C   Left monoplegia
D   Loss of pain and temperature sensation on the left side
E   Loss of proprioception and vibration sense on the left side

18. A 33-year-old man was hit on his head during a fight. He was suspected of having an extradural haematoma. Which of the following signs is the first indication of raised intracranial pressure causing compression of cranial nerve III?

A   Constriction of the ipsilateral pupil

B   Dilatation of the ipsilateral pupil
C   Ipsilateral eyeball abducted and directed slightly inferiorly
D   Ipsilateral ptosis
E   Ipsilateral slowness of the pupillary response

19. A 55-year-old man diagnosed with hypothyroidism complained that he had an aching pain in his right hand with paraesthesia, occurring mainly at night. Which sign are you most likely to elicit?

A   Ability to oppose the thumb
B   Loss of pronation of the forearm
C   No sensory loss over the palm
D   Sensory loss over the little finger
E   Wasting of the thenar muscles

20. A 70-year-old woman presented with hearing loss and tinnitus. Investigations led to a diagnosis of acoustic neuroma. You examine the patient's cranial nerves. What sign are you most likely to elicit?

A   Facial hyperaesthesia
B   Facial weakness
C   Impaired gag reflex
D   Intact corneal reflex
E   Ptosis

ASSESSMENT

21. You were called to assess an 83-year-old man who was found wandering by the police. During the MMSE, you asked him to remember three objects but he was unable to repeat them after 1 minute. Which type of memory deficit has been elicited?

A   Anterograde memory
B   Declarative memory
C   Episodic memory
D   Retrograde memory
E   Working memory

22. A 79-year-old widow with Alzheimer's disease attended the day hospital regularly. She continued enjoying knitting, which she used to do before developing her condition. Which of her memories remains intact?

A   Declarative memory
B   Episodic memory
C   Procedural memory
D   Retrograde memory
E   Semantic memory

23. A 31-year-old man was unconscious for 1 week after a road traffic accident. On examination, he had no memory for any events for a period of 2 weeks before the accident. What type of memory loss does this refer to?

A   Anterograde memory
B   Episodic memory
C   Retrograde memory
D   Semantic memory
E   Working memory

24. A 23-year-old man with schizophrenia presented with complaints of visual hallucinations, restlessness and marked thirst. On examination, he was agitated and had a raised body temperature, dilated pupils, dry mouth and urinary retention. Which of the following is most likely to account for this clinical presentation?

    A   Antimuscarinic intoxication
    B   Benzodiazepine withdrawal
    C   Catatonia
    D   Cocaine withdrawal
    E   Opioid intoxication

25. Which of the following single-photon emission computed tomography (SPECT) scan reports is characteristic of Alzheimer's disease?

    A   Increased perfusion in the frontal lobes
    B   Increased perfusion in the lateral temporal lobes
    C   Increased perfusion in the parietal lobes
    D   Reduced perfusion in the occipital lobes
    E   Reduced perfusion in the posterior temporal lobes

26. Which of the following tests is used to assess executive function?

    A   Adaptive behaviour scales
    B   Goldstein object sorting test
    C   Hayling's sentence completion test
    D   MMSE
    E   Rey–Osterrieth complex figure test

27. Which of the following is a specific test for frontal lobe dysfunction?

    A   Cognitive estimates test
    B   Digit-span task
    C   Raven's progressive matrices
    D   Repertory grid test
    E   Wechsler memory scale

ETIOLOGY

28. Polymorphism of genes is associated with an increased risk of depression when exposed to psychosocial stressors. Which of the following is affected?

    A   Dopamine D_2-receptor
    B   Dopamine transporter
    C   Monoamine oxidase A
    D   Monoamine oxidase B
    E   Serotonin transporter

29. Which of the following is a risk factor for attention deficit hyperactivity disorder?

    A   Being a first-born child
    B   High levels of homovanillic acid
    C   High levels of noradrenaline metabolites (3-methyl-4-hydrophenyl glycol)
    D   Large family size
    E   Polymorphism in the dopamine D_4 transporter gene

30. An 82-year-old widow living with her son presented with the first onset of somatic and auditory hallucinations accompanied by persecutory delusions. Which of the following is a risk factor for this presentation?

    A   Alcohol abuse
    B   Being a widow
    C   Benzodiazepine addiction
    D   HLA-DR15-DQ6
    E   Impaired hearing

31. The current evidence suggests that the risk of developing psychiatric illness is increased within 6 months of a significant life event. By what factor is this risk increased?

    A   1–2
    B   2–7
    C   7–10
    D   10–14
    E   14–20

32. With what is HLA-DQB1-*0602 mainly associated?

    A   Alzheimer's disease
    B   Huntington's disease
    C   Klein–Levin syndrome
    D   Narcolepsy
    E   Schizophrenia

33. Which of the following parts of the brain is likely to be involved in the difference between homosexual and heterosexual men?

    A   Cortex
    B   Hypothalamus
    C   Medulla
    D   Pons
    E   Thalamus

34. An 8-year-old girl frequently got into trouble at school because she disturbed the other pupils and could not sit still in the classroom. However, when she was alone with her tutor she worked well and productively. What is the most likely aetiology of this child's problem?

    A   Excessive punishment
    B   Food additives
    C   Lead exposure
    D   Neurological dysfunction
    E   Over-leniency

35. With what is tuberous sclerosis most likely to be associated?

    A   ADHD
    B   Autism
    C   Conduct disorders
    D   Encopresis
    E   Enuresis

DIAGNOSIS

36. A 25-year-old female postgraduate student became extremely angry when her college thesis committee refused to approve her project. She claimed, 'They are just jealous of me because I will be the most brilliant scientist in the United Kingdom'. It has been observed that she has had such attitudes all her life. What is the most likely diagnosis?

    A   Anxious (avoidant) personality disorder
    B   Emotionally unstable personality disorder
    C   Histrionic personality disorder
    D   Narcissistic personality disorder
    E   Passive–aggressive personality disorder

37. A 30-year-old female nurse had recurrent intrusive thoughts of stabbing a patient with a hypodermic needle. She found the thoughts unpleasant, horrible and anxiety provoking, but was able to resist them. What is the most likely diagnosis?

    A   Antisocial personality disorder
    B   Dependent personality disorder
    C   Emotionally unstable personality disorder
    D   Generalised anxiety disorder
    E   Obsessive–compulsive disorder

38. A 26-year-old man liked wearing clothes of the opposite sex. He did not get any sexual gratification from the act but just enjoyed membership of the opposite sex. There was no desire for a sex change. What is the most likely diagnosis?

    A   Dual-role transvestism
    B   Fetishistic transvestism
    C   Sadomasochism
    D   Transsexualism
    E   Voyeurism

39. An 18-year-old man presented with transient perceptual abnormalities and incongruent affect. He was noticed to be giggling to himself. There were affective changes and some evidence of a thought disorder. What is the most likely diagnosis?

    A   Catatonic schizophrenia
    B   Hebephrenic (disorganised) schizophrenia
    C   Paranoid schizophrenia
    D   Schizotypal disorder
    E   Simple schizophrenia

40. According to the *International Classification of Diseases*, 10th revision (ICD-10), which of the following is a diagnostic criterion of paranoid personality disorder?

    A   Being excessively sensitive to setbacks and rebuffs
    B   Excessive efforts to avoid abandonment
    C   Inability to experience guilt
    D   Lack of desire for close friends or confiding relationships
    E   Rigidity and stubbornness

41. On which DSM-IV (*Diagnostic and Statistical Manual of Mental Disorders*, 4th edn) axis, is a medical condition coexisting with a mental disorder recorded?

    A   Axis I only
    B   Axis III only

    C   Axis V only
    D   Axis I and axis III
    E   Axis I and axis V

42. What is the main difference between the DSM-IV-TR and the ICD-10 criteria used for the diagnosis of post-traumatic stress disorder?

    A   Avoidance
    B   Exposure to traumatic event
    C   Functional impairment
    D   Hypervigilance
    E   Reliving

43. According to the ICD-10 classification, onset of symptoms in post-traumatic stress disorder should be within a specified period of time. What is this duration?

    A   1 month
    B   3 months
    C   4 months
    D   6 months
    E   12 months

44. Which publication of the ICD had included a section on mental disorders for the first time?

    A   ICD-4
    B   ICD-5
    C   ICD-6
    D   ICD-7
    E   ICD-8

45. You get a call from the duty physician about a 38-year-old man with a bipolar affective disorder whose mental state had been stable on lithium carbonate. The duty physician would like to start him on a diuretic as soon as possible. Which of the following diuretics does not interfere with the serum concentration of lithium?

    A   Bendroflumethiazide
    B   Furosemide
    C   Indapamide
    D   Mannitol
    E   Spironolactone

46. A 45-year-old man with a family history of diabetes mellitus presented with psychotic symptoms. Which of the following antipsychotics does not interfere with blood sugar?

    A   Amisulpride
    B   Haloperidol
    C   Olanzapine
    D   Quetiapine
    E   Risperidone

47. You get a call from the duty obstetrician about a 32-year-old woman who was 15 weeks' pregnant and her bipolar affective disorder was stabilised on lithium. Which of the following statements about use of lithium in pregnancy is correct?

    A   Lithium is not excreted in breast milk.
    B   Lithium use does not affect the fetus in the second trimester
    C   Lithium use in the first trimester is associated with neural tube defects in the fetus
    D   Serum lithium levels increase in the third trimester of pregnancy
    E   Serum lithium levels increase in the immediate postpartum period

48. Which of the following mood stabilisers has the best evidence for reducing the rates of completed suicides in bipolar affective disorder?

A   Carbamazepine
B   Gabapentin
C   Lamotrigine
D   Lithium
E   Valproate

49. You review a 42-year-old man with a psychotic episode on the ward. He had been prescribed quetiapine since his admission last week. He went on leave and had a glass of grapefruit juice at home. How does grapefruit juice affect quetiapine metabolism?

A   Chemical components of grapefruit juice can free more quetiapine from protein-binding site
B   Grapefruit juice decreases the excretion of quetiapine
C   Grapefruit juice has no effect on quetiapine metabolism
D   Grapefruit juice irreversibly blocks intestinal cytochrome P450
E   Grapefruit juice reversibly blocks intestinal cytochrome P450

BASIC PSYCHOLOGICAL PROCESSES

50. A 45-year-old man wanted to stop smoking and therefore engaged himself in a therapy programme, where the act of smoking was paired with imagining a horrible taste. On every occasion thereafter, every time he got an urge to smoke, he imagined the horrible taste. This approach helped him to stop smoking.

What technique has his therapist used to help him stop smoking?

A   Aversion therapy
B   Covert sensitisation
C   Flooding
D   Implosion
E   Systemic desensitisation

51. Systemic desensitisation is an application of classic conditioning. What is the principle involved?

A   Covert sensitisation and implosion
B   Flooding and reciprocal inhibition
C   Flooding and systemic desensitisation
D   Implosion and reciprocal inhibition
E   Reciprocal inhibition and systemic desensitisation

52. Which of the following statements about assimilation in Piaget's theory of cognitive development is correct?

A   It is a process through which a child interprets new experiences by incorporating them into an existing schema
B   It is a process by which the child modifies existing schema to incorporate new experiences
C   It leads to development of new schema
D   It occurs after accommodation
E   It occurs before adaptation

53. At what age does object permanence occur?

A   6–12 months
B   12–18 months

    C   18–24 months
    D   24–30 months
    E   30–36 months

54. What do we call drawing inferences about the relationship between two things based on a single shared attribute?

    A   Conservation
    B   Egocentricism
    C   Hypothetico-deductive reasoning
    D   Object permanence
    E   Transductive reasoning

55. Which of the following occurs in the sensorimotor stage of Piaget's theory of cognitive development?

    A   Animism
    B   Conservation
    C   Egocentrism
    D   Reflex activity
    E   Transductive reasoning

56. Which of the following statements about Piaget's stages of cognitive development is correct?

    A   In the sensorimotor stage, the child is egocentric
    B   Lack of conservation is a feature of the formal operational stage
    C   Logical reasoning is not present until the formal operational stage
    D   Non-logical thought is a feature of children aged 7–11 years
    E   The preoperational stage lasts for about 5 years

57. Which of the behavioural theorists first described the concept of operant conditioning?

    A   Kohlberg
    B   Pavlov
    C   Piaget
    D   Seligman
    E   Skinner

58. An 8-month-old girl enjoyed picking up toys and bringing them to her mouth. She was often seen sucking them. What phase of Freud's psychosexual development is she going through?

    A   Anal phase
    B   Genital phase
    C   Latency phase
    D   Oral phase
    E   Phallic phase

59. According to Freud, during psychosexual development a boy focuses his love on his mother. This can reach a stage where a boy becomes jealous of his father and wants to kill him. However, he cannot do this for fear of castration and so represses these urges as he moves to the next stage of development. Which of the following describes the boy's psychosocial development?

    A   Anal phase
    B   Genital phase
    C   Latency phase
    D   Oedipus complex
    E   Phallic phase

60. A child copies a circle, uses basic grammatically correct sentences, shows cooperative play, has a fear of animals and the dark, and also has his own sexual identity. What is his age?

    A   2 years
    B   3 years
    C   4 years
    D   5 years
    E   6 years

61. A 24-year-old man exhibited an outpouring of emotions during a lengthy discussion of childhood memories. He was often angry, rambled excessively, and was distressed and tearful. Which category of Mary Main's adult attachment interview is he representing?

    A   Deprivation
    B   Dismissing
    C   Disorganised
    D   Preoccupied/Entangled
    E   Secure/Autonomous

62. A child encountered a horse for the first time and called it a 'doggie'. What is the term developed by Jean Piaget for this cognitive process?

    A   Adaptation
    B   Accommodation
    C   Assimilation
    D   Equilibration
    E   Schemas

63. At which stage of Margaret Mahler's theory of cognitive development does a child perceive his or he mother and self as one unit?

    A   Autism
    B   Differentiation
    C   Object constancy
    D   Practising
    E   Symbiosis

64. With what is Lawrence Kohlberg associated?

    A   Cognitive reasoning in adults
    B   Description of the four major stages of morality
    C   Description of the good mother
    D   Extension of Mary Main's theory of cognitive development in children
    E   Moral reasoning in adults

65. Which of the following statements about catharsis is correct?

    A   It is always necessary to discharge or reduce aggression
    B   Catharsis is most unlikely to be associated with aggression
    C   It is most effective in the management of violent behaviour
    D   It leads to more aggression in patients undergoing catharsis
    E   It is predominantly effective in the long-term management of aggression

66. In which stage of cognitive development, are phenomenalistic causality and animistic thinking are seen?

    A   Concrete operational
    B   Concrete sensorimotor
    C   Formal operational

D   Preoperational
E   Presensorimotor

SOCIAL PSYCHOLOGY

67. A 21-year-old woman always felt that she was not as good as her older sister. Which one of
     Argyle's four dimensions does the above describe?

A   Ego-strength
B   Integration of the self
C   Self-esteem
D   Self-image
E   The ego-ideal

68. Teachers tend to take the credit for a student's academic success but will attribute a student's
     poor performance to his or her laziness. Which of the following describes the 'fundamental
     attribution error'?

A   He failed the examination because he did not have enough time to finish his paper
B   He failed the examination because he did not study hard enough
C   He failed the examination due to the ambiguous questions set by the examiners
D   He passed the examination due to my hard work and academic prowess
E   He failed the examination because the exam hall was too noisy

69. French and Raven described the social power derived from the ability to allocate resources. What
     is this called?

A   Authority
B   Coercive
C   Expert
D   Referent
E   Reward

70. Which of the following increases prejudice?

A   Cooperative effort
B   Equal status
C   Exposure to non-stereotypical individual
D   Social environment favouring equality
E   Stereotyping of the victim of prejudice

DESCRIPTION AND MEASUREMENT

71. What does the valid test of orientation in a 25-year-old delirious patient include?

A   Ability to perform mental arithmetic
B   Awareness of the role of the interviewer
C   Giving correct date of birth
D   Giving correct information about their family
E   Giving current address

72. Which of the following statements about the serial sevens test is correct?

A   It is a bedside diagnostic test of Alzheimer's disease
B   It is a good indicator of concentration

C   It can differentiate cognitive impairment due to a variety of reasons
D   It is impaired in a psychotic patient
E   It serves as an indicator of the patient's mathematical ability

73. Which of the following statements about Kelly's personal construct theory is correct?

A   It forms the basis of a therapy that aims to help people construct more effective interpretations and theories of the world
B   We are unable to develop constructs in order to deal with all kinds of situation or events in later life
C   We are unable to identify invalid theories that hinder us in later life
D   We can construct our lives or reconstruct the progress in our lives, following our impulses
E   We can engage in unconscious mental activities and consequently know about ourselves and the world

BASIC PSYCHOLOGICAL TREATMENTS

74. A 35-year-old man with alcohol problem undergoes a psychological assessment. He was now willing to accept positive advice for change, make plans for behaviour change, set goals and assess past successes and failures. At which of Prochaska and Diclemente's (1993) stages of behaviour is he at present?

A   Awareness
B   Contemplation
C   Preparation
D   Ready for action
E   Termination

75. A 15-year-old girl told you that she had been repeatedly sexually abused by her stepfather. Which is the first-line management step that you should take?

A   Cognitive–analytic therapy
B   Cognitive–behavioural therapy
C   Post-traumatic debriefing
D   Refer to social services
E   Systemic family therapy

76. A 59-year-old man presented complaining bitterly that he had recently been diagnosed with a malignancy. During the assessment, he objected to the statement that he led a healthy lifestyle. Which of the following describes this situation?

A   Emotional reasoning
B   Fallacy of fairness
C   Mental filtering
D   Reductionism
E   Self-righteous cognition

77. A 23-year-old female graduate was assessed for cognitive–behavioural therapy for generalised anxiety disorder. According to the cognitive therapy of anxiety, which of the following is correct?

A   Anxiety is a disorder of thinking
B   Anxiety is associated with hyperarousal
C   Anxiety is associated with physical symptoms
D   Catastrophisation is a major mechanism
E   Sensitisation is an essential mechanism

78. A 28-year-old single man had been taking crack cocaine for a few years. He attended a drug advisory centre at the request of his girlfriend. He did not consider this a problem and believed that his girlfriend's worries were excessive. Which of Prochaska and Diclemente's stages of change is reflected here?

   A   Preaction
   B   Precontemplation
   C   Predecision
   D   Pre-evaluation
   E   Premotivation

BASIC PSYCHOPHARMACOLOGY

79. Which of the following statements about benzodiazepine receptors is correct?

   A   Benzodiazepine receptors are associated with excitatory neurotransmitters
   B   Chlormethiazole binds to the same site as benzodiazepines
   C   These receptors are linked to sodium channels
   D   Zolpidem binds to a subtype benzodiazepine receptor-1
   E   Zopiclone binds to same site as benzodiazepines

80. Which of the following statements about lithium is correct?

   A   Lithium blood samples are taken 18 hours after last dose
   B   Only concentrations > 2.0 mmol/L are associated with an increased risk of toxicity
   C   Regular monitoring can lead to poor compliance
   D   Serum lithium concentrations should be measured with changing renal function
   E   Target lithium concentrations range between 0.1 and 0.2 mmol/L

81. Pharmacokinetic interactions occur when one drug interferes with the actions of another drug during absorption, distribution and elimination. Which of the following statements is correct?

   A   Cytochrome 450 allows psychotropic metabolism
   B   Diuretics alter the availability of lithium
   C   Monoamine oxidase inhibitors increase the metabolism of dietary amines
   D   Paracetamol reduces absorption of amitriptyline by about 50%
   E   Valproate is displaced from protein-binding sites by phenytoin

82. Which of the following statements about treatment of depressive illness without psychotic symptoms is correct?

   A   Antidepressants are effective in 90% of patients
   B   Antidepressants are effective in only 50% of patients
   C   Failure of adequate trials occurs in 25% of patients
   D   Failure of adequate trial of an antidepressant occurs in 15% of patients
   E   Nearly 60% of the partial responders to antidepressants benefit from addition of lithium

83. Which of the following statements about the adverse effects of lithium is correct?

   A   10–20% of patients show morphological kidney changes with long-term therapy
   B   After 6–18 months of treatment, 60% of women develop hypothyroidism
   C   More than 10% of patients develop irreversible kidney failure after 10 years of treatment
   D   The estimated risk of major congenital abnormalities for lithium-exposed babies is 80%
   E   Up to 70% of patients treated with lithium experience side effects

84. Which of the following statements about regarding the sedative property of tricyclic and tetracyclic antidepressants is correct?

   A   Amitriptyline is the least sedating tricyclic antidepressant
   B   Desipramine is the most sedating tricyclic antidepressant
   C   Tetracyclic antidepressants have a sedative effect due to anticholinergic properties
   D   Trazodone is a highly sedative tetracyclic antidepressant
   E   Tricyclic antidepressants have a sedative effect due to 5-hydroxytryptamine (5-HT$_2$) antagonism

85. A 57-year-old man with hypertension, myocardial infarction and depression received treatment with fluoxetine. However, he developed severe hyponatraemia. Which of the following medications is most suitable in this case for the treatment of depression?

   A   Citalopram
   B   Mirtazapine
   C   Quetiapine
   D   Reboxetine
   E   Sertraline

86. In the treatment of bipolar depression, the National Institute for Health and Care Excellence (NICE) recommends the use of quetiapine, provided that it satisfies one of the following criteria. What is that criterion?

   A   An antimanic agent has not been prescribed
   B   An antimanic has already been prescribed
   C   An antipsychotic and antimanic have not been previously tried
   D   An antipsychotic has already been prescribed
   E   An antipsychotic has not been prescribed

87. In the treatment of post-stroke depression of a patient who is also taking warfarin, which of the following is the most suitable antidepressant?

   A   Citalopram
   B   Dapoxetine
   C   Fluoxetine
   D   Fluvoxamine
   E   Paroxetine

PREVENTION OF PSYCHIATRIC DISORDERS

88. A 17-year-old man presented to the outpatient clinic with symptoms suggestive of psychosis. He reported having smoked cannabis on a regular basis since a young age. Which of the following statements about cannabis and onset of psychosis is correct?

   A   Age of onset of psychosis is 2.7 years earlier in cannabis users
   B   Alcohol use is linked with a younger age of onset of psychosis
   C   Cannabis does not influence the age of onset of psychosis
   D   Cannabis users have a delayed onset of psychosis
   E   Cannabis is the only illicit drug linked with an earlier onset of psychosis

89. A 27-year-old man has recovered from his first episode of psychosis. His family does not want him to take medication for 'longer than is needed' due to side effects. Which of the following statements about the first 5 years after the onset of a first episode of psychosis is correct?

   A   Most patients who experience a single episode of psychosis never relapse after remission

B   Up to half of patients who experience a first episode psychosis relapse within 3 years of remission

C   Up to half of patients who experience a first episode psychosis relapse within 5 years of remission

D   Up to 20% of patients who experience a first episode psychosis relapse within 5 years of remission

E   Up to 80% of patients who experience a first episode psychosis relapse within 5 year of remission

90. Which of the following statements about childhood abuse is correct?

A   Boys experience more physical abuse than girls
B   Boys experience more sexual abuse than girls
C   Fathers are more likely to physically abuse their children
D   Mothers are more likely to sexually abuse their children
E   Mothers are as likely as fathers to sexually abuse their children

DESCRIPTIVE PSYCHOPATHOLOGY

91. Which of the following is an example of sensory deception?

A   Derealisation
B   Increased sensitivity to noise
C   Perceived irregularity of the shape of an object
D   Seeing vivid pictures in clouds
E   Yellow colouring of visual perception

92. Which of the following is a sensory distortion?

A   Dysmegalopsia
B   Hallucinosis
C   Pareidolia
D   Phantom limb
E   Synaesthesia

93. Which of the following statements about illusions is correct?

A   Affect illusions are clinically different from hallucinations
B   Auditory illusions are the most common modality of illusions
C   Illusions do not occur in delirium
D   Illusions in themselves indicate of psychopathology
E   Pareidolia consists of vivid illusions without any extra effort

94. Which of the following statements about hallucinations is correct?

A   Charles Bonnet syndrome includes clouding of consciousness
B   Hallucinations are pathognomonic of psychotic disorders
C   Hallucinosis is a characteristic feature of alcohol intoxication
D   Lesions of the diencephalon can lead to auditory hallucinations
E   Normal people can be persuaded to hallucinate

95. A 24-year-old man smelt burning rubber when he saw red signal at traffic lights and was convinced of the link between them. What is this phenomenon known as?

A   Extracampine hallucination
B   Functional hallucination

C   Primary delusion
D   Reflex hallucination
E   Sensory distortion

96. A 45-year-old man has been diagnosed as having locked-in syndrome. Which of the following statements is correct?

A   All the muscles are paralysed
B   It is caused by a lesion in motor pathways in the dorsal pons
C   It is characterised by akinetic mutism
D   Consciousness is clouded
E   Joints in the arms and legs get locked, leading to rigidity

97. A 69-year-old woman was found wandering in the streets. She was disoriented on assessment in the accident and emergency department. Which of the following statements about orientation is correct?

A   Disorientation rules out a functional psychiatric illness
B   Established disorientation in time and place requires clouding of consciousness
C   Hysterical dissociation is present with apparent disorientation
D   Loss of the knowledge of the patient's own name and identity occurs before the disorientation of others' identity
E   Orientation in space is disturbed before orientation in time

98. A 52-year-old man with a long history of alcohol dependence and memory problems presents with confabulation. Which one of the following is correct with regard to confabulation?

A   Memory of actual events displaced in space or time
B   Diagnostic feature of Korsakoff's syndrome
C   False memory syndrome as the memory is impaired
D   Effects on autobiographical memory rare
E   Patient aware of memory deficits

99. Which of the following is pathognomonic of organic brain disease?

A   Amnesia
B   Confabulation
C   Confusion
D   Disorientation
E   Perseveration

100. A 24-year-old man suddenly collapsed on hearing the news of his country winning the world cup. What is the most likely phenomenon?

A   Catalepsy
B   Cataplexy
C   Catatonia
D   Dissociative paralysis
E   Sleep paralysis

101. A 21-year-old man saw a car flashing its indicator to turn right and immediately believed that he was the heir to the throne. What is this phenomenon called?

A   Delusions of grandeur
B   Misidentification syndrome
C   Primary delusion
D   Reflex hallucination
E   Secondary delusion

102. A 26-year-old woman believed that she was the owner of the Manchester United Football Club. Which of the following dimensions best describes the severity of the delusion?

   A   Content
   B   Diagnosis
   C   Duration
   D   Frequency
   E   Pressure

103. A patient says 'I am well today-ay-ay-ay-ay...'. What is this an example of?

   A   Automatic obedience
   B   Echolalia
   C   Echopraxia
   D   Logoclonia
   E   Stuttering

104. You administered the MMSE to a 65-year-old man. On asking about the day of the week, he said 'Monday'. Then you asked him about the month and he still said 'Monday'. When you asked him about the year, he told you 'Monday'. What is this best described as?

   A   Automatism
   B   Mannerism
   C   Perseveration
   D   Stereotypy
   E   Stuttering

105. Which of the following is a characteristic feature of depersonalisation?

   A   Affect can be pleasant in some cases
   B   Ego boundaries get dissolved
   C   Insight is often impaired
   D   It is a subjective experience
   E   It is clearly distinguishable from derealisation

106. What does the 'serial sevens' test assess?

   A   Attention
   B   Concentration
   C   Executive functions
   D   Orientation
   E   Retention

107. A doctor, when carrying out a physical examination of the cardiovascular system on a female patient, asked her to unbutton her 'skirt' instead of her 'shirt'. What is this described as?

   A   Logoclonia
   B   Neologism
   C   Paragrammatism
   D   Parapraxis
   E   Stock word

108. What is Broca's dysphasia characterised by?

   A   Conduction aphasia
   B   Fluent aphasia
   C   Scanning speech
   D   Staccato speech
   E   Telegraphic speech

109. Which of following is not an extreme form of cooperation?

    A   Advertence
    B   Echopraxia
    C   *Gegenhalten*
    D   *Mitgehen*
    E   *Mitmachen*

110. What is familiarity with an unfamiliar situation called?

    A   Déjà-vu
    B   Jamais-vu
    C   Recognition
    D   Recollection
    E   Retrieval

111. Which of the following explains memory impairment accurately?

    A   Confabulation is an example of a problem with 'retention'
    B   Following a cerebral trauma, retrograde amnesia occurs due to problems in registration
    C   In Korsakoff's syndrome, memory impairment occurs due to a problem in recall
    D   Memory impairment due to electroconvulsive therapy includes apparent loss of memory stores
    E   Memory stays intact in a fugue state

112. According to the Kübler–Ross model, which of the following constitutes one of the stages of grief?

    A   Anger
    B   Anxiety
    C   Flashbacks
    D   Insomnia
    E   Mourning

113. A 35-year-old man believed that this world was a dirty place to live in. He washed his hands several times and took a bath twice a day. He drank only bottled water, washed his clothes in hot water with a particular detergent, got medically examined every 6 months and stayed away from pets. He does not think that there is anything wrong in such thinking. Which of the following describes the psychopathology?

    A   Delusion of contamination
    B   No psychopathology
    C   Obsession and compulsion
    D   Overvalued idea
    E   Specific phobia of contamination

DYNAMIC PSYCHOPATHOLOGY

114. A 22-year-old medical student, confronted with an enormous mass of information and responsibility, became engrossed in her work, and felt less anxious and mentally stronger for continuing her studies. Which of the following coping mechanisms can explain the situation?

    A   Denial
    B   Humour
    C   Mastery and control
    D   Reaction formation
    E   Sublimation

115. During an individual psychotherapy session, the therapist began talking excessively and confronted the patient. This was probably a result of something in the patient's behaviour and his interaction with the therapist. What is this an example of?

    A   Countertransference
    B   Displacement
    C   Projection
    D   Projective identification
    E   Transference

HISTORY OF PSYCHIATRY

116. Who was associated with replacing 'dementia praecox' by the term 'schizophrenia'?

    A   Adolf Mayer
    B   Eugen Bleuler
    C   Kahlbaum
    D   Kraepelin
    E   Schneider

117. Who was responsible for translating 'démence précoce' into 'dementia praecox'?

    A   Adolf Mayer
    B   Eugen Bleuler
    C   Kahlbaum
    D   Kraepelin
    E   Schneider

118. Who coined the term 'démence précoce'?

    A   Adolf Mayer
    B   Eugen Bleuler
    C   Kahlbaum
    D   Kraepelin
    E   Morel

119. In 1983, Raven developed Raven's progressive matrices test to overcome which of the following limitations of previous tests?

    A   Age bias in IQ testing
    B   Blindness while IQ testing
    C   Cultural bias in IQ testing
    D   Language bias in IQ testing
    E   Racial bias in IQ testing

120. What does Plutchik's wheel represent?

    A   Emotions
    B   Intelligence
    C   Memory
    D   Perception
    E   Personality

121. Who is associated with the concept of 'good-enough mothers'?

    A   Ainsworth
    B   Bowlby

C   Harlow
D   Mahler
E   Winnicott

122. Which of the following statements about Freud's 'interpretation of dreams' is correct?

A   Dream work is the process by which unconscious wishes are processed into dreams
B   Secondary revision refers to dreams that recur time and again
C   Dreams are manifestations of unconscious fears
D   The manifest content is not accessible to the dreamer
E   The latent content of the dreams refers to the meaning behind them

123. Which of the following is credited to Benedict Morel?

A   Described bizarre symptoms in hebephrenia
B   Described schizophrenia in people with an 'asthenic' body type
C   Described 'true schizophrenia'
D   Differentiated patients with schizophrenia and manic–depressive psychosis
E   Using the term '*démence précoce*'

BASIC ETHICS AND PHILOSOPHY OF PSYCHIATRY

124. Which of the following statements about the findings of International pilot study of schizophrenia is correct?

A   Catatonic symptoms were frequent among patients in developing countries
B   Delusions and hallucinations were more frequent in western populations
C   Standardised assessment and diagnostic measures were not applicable to all populations
D   The core symptoms of schizophrenia varied across cultures
E   Two-year outcome was better in developed centres

125. Which of the following statements about the cultural phenomenon of psychosis is correct?

A   At the 2-year follow-up, patients from developed countries were better
B   Incidence of core schizophrenia showed a three fold difference across centres
C   Psychotic experiences in mania are more common in Europeans than African–Caribbean patients
D   The broad diagnosis of schizophrenia (lacking schneiderian symptoms) showed a three fold difference across countries
E   The incidence of mania is the same in ethnic minorities living in developed countries as that of their native populations

126. Which of the following statements about the strange situation procedure is correct?

A   Sixty-five per cent of infants securely are attached by 12 months
B   Assessment can be done in adolescence
C   This procedure was developed by Winnicott
D   The infant is exposed to escalating amounts of stress
E   Its protocol has six steps

Answers: MCQs

1. B Circular question

Questions that are used in clinical interviews can be either facilitative or obstructive. Open questions reflect on a topic that the interviewer may want to explore but leaves it open to the patient to say what is important. Circular questioning can be confusing and obstructive in eliciting information. Closed questions will lead to a simple yes, no or a single actual answer. Put-down questions are where the underlying message is a criticism.

2. B Hypothetical question

This type of question leads to an imaginative or unspoken response in the therapy sessions. Run-on or polythematic questioning refers to the process of asking the patient a number of questions simultaneously. Interpretations are inferences reached by examining patterns of behaviour or thoughts that are expressed during a clinical session.

3. D Functional hallucination

In this type of hallucination, the presence of another real sensory modality is required. An extracampine hallucination refers to a hallucination that occurs outside the limits of the sensory field. Anxious foreboding is defined as a fear that something terrible will happen, although the person cannot identify what he or she is frightened of. It is accompanied by physical symptoms of anxiety and must be distinguished from understandable foreboding, such as that experienced by a person awaiting an interview result. An affect illusion arises in the context of a particular mood state. Kinaesthetic hallucination affects the muscles and limbs, and the patient feels that his or her limbs are being twisted, pulled or moved.

4. E Reflex hallucination

This is a form of synaesthesia which is the experience of a stimulus of one sensory modality producing a sensory experience in another. Hemisomatognosis is a unilateral lack of body image, in which the person behaves as if one side of the body is missing. It occurs in migraine or during an epileptic aura. Hyperschemazia is a perceived magnification of body parts which can occur in a variety of organic conditions such as multiple sclerosis, Brown–Séquard paralysis and blockage of the posterior inferior cerebellar artery, as well as psychiatric conditions such as hypochondriasis, depersonalisation and conversion disorders. Hyposchemazia is the diminished perception of body parts and it occurs in parietal lobe lesions such as thrombosis of the right middle cerebral artery. Paraschemazia is a feeling that parts of the body are distorted, twisted or separated from the rest of the body. It can occur in association with hallucinogenic use, epileptic aura or migraine.

5. C Lilliputian hallucinations

This is a form of visual hallucinations in which the affected person sees tiny people or objects. They may be accompanied by pleasure and amusement. Hypnagogic hallucinations occur when the person is falling asleep. It has been suggested that hypnopompic hallucinations are often hypnagogic experiences that occur in the morning when the person is waking and dosing off again, so that they actually happen when the person is falling asleep. Both hypnagogic and hypnopompic phenomena are not indicative of any psychopathology, even though they are true hallucinatory experiences. Pareidolia occurs when people see vivid pictures in fire or clouds without any conscious effort on their part and sometimes against their will.

6. A Have you been sleeping well?'

A closed question usually has a straightforward 'yes' or 'no' answer or a single word or short phrase. This form of question is helpful when obtaining a specific piece of information.

Examples of types of questions:

Polythematic question: 'How is your sleep and appetite?'

Open question: 'What brought you to the emergency department today?'

Leading statement: 'You were not sleeping at that time?'

Summarising statement: 'So, do I understand this correctly that … .'

7. D Language understanding

A three-stage command is used to test language understanding. In this part of the test, the patient is given a piece of paper and instructed to take it in the right hand, fold it in half and put it on the floor. One point is scored for each part that is done correctly. Concentration is tested by serial sevens or spelling world backwards. Recall is the part of the test when a patient is asked to repeat the three words that were used in registration. In language naming, the patient is shown a wrist watch and a pencil and asked to name these objects one after another. Verbal fluency can be tested by repetition of 'no ifs', 'ands' or 'buts'.

8. D Facial hypomimia

In Parkinson's disease, initial symptoms are tremors and bradykinesia. A patient usually complains of stiffness and aches in the limbs and joints. Fine movements are difficult to execute. Writing becomes small (micrographia) and spidery, with a tendency to tail off at the end of a line. There is a loss of arm swinging. A resting tremor of 4–7 Hz is characteristic of Parkinson's disease. The frequency of spontaneous blinking is reduced and described as a serpentine stare. The principal psychiatric consequences of this disease are depression and cognitive impairment. When stiffness is combined with tremor, smooth 'lead-pipe' rigidity is broken up into a jerky resistance to passive movement, known as cogwheel rigidity.

9. C Raven's progressive matrices

The Stanford–Binet and Wechsler scales are administered as a series of tests of different abilities. Each test is presented as a graded series of similar tasks. The MMSE is used to assess cognitive function, whereas the NART assesses the ability to read and pronounce irregular words, such as 'bouquet', and has been found to be relatively resistant to the effects of brain damage.

10. C Scores of < 82 predict dementia with 100% sensitivity

Addenbrooke's cognitive examination is an answer tool designed for routine clinical use. It assesses memory, fluency and language more comprehensively.

11. B Comprehension

Attention and concentration are tested by 'serial sevens test' or asking the patient to recite the months of the year backwards. As a result of the familiarity, errors are more likely to reflect clinically significant disorder. Orientation tends to be compromised progressively. Only 'time' is affected in mild cognitive disorder, followed by 'place', with 'person' disrupted only in severe cases. Insight generally refers to patients' ability to accept that they are ill and their willingness to accept medical recommendations.

12. B Phonemic paraphasia

In paraphasias, words are replaced. It could be semantic paraphasia or phonemic paraphasia. In phonemic paraphasia words with a similar sound are replaced, whereas in semantic paraphasia words with a similar meaning are replaced.

13. B Cactus and camel test

Tests for semantic memory include:

I.   Components from the Wechsler adult intelligence scale
II. Similarities
III. Category fluency test
IV. Object-naming test
V.   Word-to-picture match
VI. Non-verbal test picture to picture test

14. C Priming

This is an example of implicit memory. The exposure to test stimuli increases subsequent response. In the word stem completion test, patients are shown a set of words. Then, they are asked to list the words that they can remember. The last step of this test involves showing the person the first three letters of the list of words, and then asking for completion of the stem from the list of words. For example:

Step 1: patient is shown 'elephant, apple and table', etc.
Step 2: patient is asked to list the words that he or she can recall
Step 3: patient is shown 'ele..., app..., tab...', etc.
Step 4: patient is asked to complete the stems.

Amnestic patients do well on the completing task, whereas they have difficulty recalling the words later on.

15. A Frontal lobe

The Iowa gambling task is a psychological test for decision-making skills. It tests the frontal lobes.

16. E T10

This question tests knowledge of dermatomes.

Key dermatomes to remember include T4 = line of nipples (male), T10 = umbilicus, T12 = into groin.

17. D Loss of pain and temperature sensation on the left side

In the Brown–Séquard syndrome, there is spastic weakness and loss of proprioception and vibration sense on the side ipsilateral to the lesion. There is loss of pain and temperature sensation in the contralateral side to the lesion.

18. E Ipsilateral slowness of the pupillary response

As intracranial pressure rises, cranial nerve III is compressed against the crest of the petrous part of the temporal bone. As autonomic fibres are the most superficial they are first to be affected, leading to ipsilateral slowness of the pupillary response to light.

19. E Wasting of the thenar muscles

This is a case of carpal tunnel syndrome. Compression of the median nerve at the wrist leads to paralysis and wasting of the thenar muscles (excluding adductor pollicis) and the radial two lumbrical muscles. There is a loss of sensation over the thumb, adjacent two half-fingers and over the radial two-thirds of the palm. If the median nerve is divided at the elbow, then pronation of the forearm is lost, and wrist flexion is weak and accompanied by ulnar deviation.

20. B Facial weakness

This is a case of a cerebellopontine angle syndrome. The cerebellopontine angle is a triangle between the lateral pons, cerebellum and petrous bone, into which cranial nerves V–VIII emerge. Acoustic neuromas may lead to signs corresponding to compression of these nerves. Likely signs seen are nystagmus, loss of facial sensation, facial weakness and loss of corneal reflex.

21. E Working memory

This is another name for short-term memory. It is an active workbench for carrying out mental operations such as simple mathematical calculations (e.g. additions, subtractions) and other cognitive operations. Episodic memory contains memory for specific episodes in life. It is also sometimes known as autobiographical memory. Declarative memory is any memory that one can bring to mind and is often, although not necessarily, capable of being spoken.

22. C Procedural memory

This is also called non-declarative memory. Examples of procedural memory include knowledge of how to ride a bike, how to swim and how to drive or write. By their very nature, procedural memories are hard to pass on to others because the information cannot be brought to mind and verbalised.

23. C Retrograde memory

Amnesia refers to a loss of memory. Retrograde amnesia is the loss of episodic memories that were stored before the brain damage. Anterograde amnesia is the inability to form or retain new episodic memories. Semantic memory includes memory for the facts, general knowledge and meaning of words.

24. A Antimuscarinic intoxication

Antimuscarinic drugs such as orphenadrine, procyclidine and trihexyphenidyl exert their anti-parkinsonian action by reducing the effects of relative central cholinergic excess which occurs as a result of dopamine deficiency. They should be used with caution in cardiovascular disease, hypertension, prostatic hypertrophy and pyrexia, in those susceptible to angle-closure glaucoma and in elderly people.

25. E Reduced perfusion in the posterior temporal lobes

In a vast majority of patients with an established diagnosis of Alzheimer's disease, structural imaging is generally non-contributory. Since the emergence of SPECT, the functional changes in the brain can be detected earlier. SPECT studies in Alzheimer's disease show diminished blood flow in the posterior temporal and inferior cortices, with temporal changes predicting mild cognitive impairment and Alzheimer's disease in healthy elderly people. Similar changes can be detected with functional magnetic resonance imaging (fMRI) and MR spectroscopy .

26. C Hayling's sentence completion test

This test provides a measure of initiation speed as well as performance on a response suppression task. It taps particular behaviours that are commonly exhibited by patients following frontal lobe damage.

27. A Cognitive estimates test

This test requires the participants to give educated guesses to questions to which they are unlikely to know the exact answers, e.g. 'How fast do race horses gallop? What is the age of the oldest person in Britain today?' Responses are scored in terms of extremes from 0 (normal) to 3 (very normal).

28. E Serotonin transporter

The monoamine theory of depression suggests that allelic variation in genes coding for monoamine synthesis or metabolism or specific receptors may contribute to the risk of mood disorders. There is some evidence that variation in the serotonin transporter gene is associated with mood disorders and also with the trait of neuroticism, a risk factor for depression.

29. E Polymorphism in the dopamine D_4 transporter gene

Linkage studies have reported an association between attention deficit hyperactivity disorder and the dopamine D_4-receptor gene and with an allele of the dopamine transporter gene. These findings are consistent with evidence that drugs affecting the dopamine system lead to improvement in the disorder. Attention deficit hyperactivity disorder is frequent among young children living in poor social conditions.

30. E Impaired hearing

Late paraphrenia or late-onset schizophrenia does not have a clear and unequivocal place in either the ICD-10 or the DSM-IV. A number of aetiological factors have emerged and include conduct deafness, poor premorbid adjustment, indicated by lower marriage and child-bearing rates. The risk of schizophrenia in first-degree relatives of these patients is 3.4% compared with 5.8% in relatives of young schizophrenia patients.

31. B 2–7

The magnitude of the effect of life events on the causation of psychiatric illness, using the general population as a control, consistently indicates risks of illness increased by factors of between two and seven in the 6-month period after an event. The risks are greater for depression and neuroses than for schizophrenia, and even greater for suicide attempts. In general, the importance of life events in the onset of a depressive episode decreases as the number of episodes increases.

32. D Narcolepsy

The narcolepsy prevalence is 5 per 10,000. It is associated with HLA-DQB-1*0602, which is present in over 85% of cases in some families with apparent autosomal transmission, compared with 18–35% in the general population. The linkage studies provided evidence that loci on 6p, 8p and 22q are associated with schizophrenia.

33. B Hypothalamus

According to the research conducted by S Le Vay, there is a difference in the structure of the hypothalamus of homosexual and heterosexual men. Postpartum tissues of heterosexual men and women were measured and compared with those of with homosexual men. Interstitial nuclei of the anterior hypothalamus were measured. It was found that the volume of interstitial nuclei of the anterior hypothalamus in heterosexual men is more than twice that of homosexual men and heterosexual women.

34. D Neurological dysfunction

The aetiology of attention deficit hyperactivity disorder is multifactorial, with genetic, functional metabolism impairment of the frontal lobe, dopamine and noradrenaline dysregulation in the prefrontal cortex, as well as psychosocial issues such as poor attachment or family dysfunction.

35. B Autism

Autism is associated with Down's syndrome, fragile X syndrome, maternal rubellar infection and tuberous sclerosis.

36. D Narcissistic personality disorder

The characteristic features of narcissistic personality disorder include grandiosity, lack of empathy, and a need for admiration. It is more common in men than in women. Its prevalence is under 1% in the general population and 2–16% in outpatient and inpatient settings. It is frequently associated with borderline, histrionic, paranoid and antisocial personality disorders. These patients frequently have vulnerable self-esteem. Their criticism frequently results in feelings of humiliation or emptiness which they do not display outwardly. They may counteract with rage, disdain or sarcasm.

37. E Obsessive–compulsive disorder

In the ICD-10, obsessive–compulsive disorder (OCD) is described under neurotic, stress-related disorders. OCD is characterised by obsessions and compulsions that are present for a period of 2 weeks. It can be in the form of thoughts or acts that are compulsive. Thoughts are repetitive, intrusive and persistent, and don't make any sense to the person who has them. The thoughts are present with anxiety and are ego-dystonia. OCD can present with repetitive acts such as washing, cleaning and counting. These acts are performed to neutralise the thoughts or doubts and are not enjoyed by the person.

38. A Dual-role transvestism

There are two types of transvestism: dual-role and fetishistic transvestism. In dual-role transvestism, the person wants to wear clothes of the opposite gender just to get temporary membership of the group, with no sexual gratification. In fetishistic transvestism, the sexual activity is principally for sexual excitement and to copy the appearance of the opposite sex. This can be the earlier phase leading to transsexualism.

39. B Hebephrenic (disorganised) schizophrenia

This type of schizophrenia occurs in late adolescence interfering with the thought processes, hence causing thought disorder. There is a prominent affective component with incongruent affect. The perceptual abnormalities and delusions are transient. The average age onset of paranoid schizophrenia is 21 years for men and 26 years for women, with equal prevalence. In simple schizophrenia, there are no obvious psychotic symptoms; there is in fact social withdrawal with academic decline.

40. A Being excessively sensitive to setbacks and rebuffs

Other features of paranoid personality disorder include unforgiving of insults, suspiciousness, and a tendency to distort experience by misconstruing the neutral or friendly actions of others as hostile or contemptuous and recurrent suspicions without justification. Excessive efforts to avoid abandonment are a feature of emotionally unstable personality disorder. C and D are features of dissocial personality disorder. Rigidity and stubbornness are features of anankastic or obsessional personality disorder.

41. D Axis I and Axis III

The DSM-IV is a multi-axial classification system. Axis I describes clinical disorders and other related illness. Axis III lists general medical conditions that may be present in addition to a mental disorder. However, when a mental disorder is caused by a general medical condition – it is listed on axis I. A general medical condition is listed on both axis I and axis III.

According to an example in the DSM-IV-TR: in a patient with depression due to hypothyroidism

Axis I: mood disorder/depression due to hypothyroidism (general medical condition)

Axis III: hypothyroidism (general medical condition)

42. C Functional impairment

Although the ICD-10 and the DSM-IV-TR criteria for diagnosis of post-traumatic stress disorder are similar, there are some differences. One of the main differences is that the ICD-10 does not specify functional impairment criteria, as does the DSM-IV-TR.

43. D 6 months

According to the ICD-10 classification, symptoms of post-traumatic stress disorder (PTSD) must be met within 6 months of the stressful event or of the end of period of stress. In some cases, onset of symptoms after 6 months can be considered, but would need to be documented and a reason given. The ICD-10 does not mention for how long the symptoms should continue before a diagnosis can be made. The criteria just mention the onset of symptoms and not their duration or length.

According to the DSM-IV-TR, symptoms of PTSD should continue for a month before the diagnosis can be made. However, it does not indicate any criteria for duration of onset of symptoms.

44. C ICD-6

In 1948, for the first time a section on mental disorders was included in ICD-6. However, the ICD-6 and the subsequent ICD-7 included only names and code numbers and were not widely used for clinical purpose.

45. B Furosemide

Thiazide diuretics, i.e. bendroflumethiazide and indapamide, reduce renal lithium clearance and increase the serum concentration. Hence toxicity might occur. Osmotic diuretics increase renal clearance of lithium, and hence decrease serum lithium concentration. Spironolactone is a potassium-sparing diuretic. It may increase serum lithium concentration. Loop diuretics usually do not affect lithium clearance, and so may be used.

46. A Amisulpride

Hyperglycaemia has been reported with haloperidol. Olanzapine, risperidone and quetiapine are associated with impaired glucose tolerance, diabetes and diabetic ketoacidosis. Amisulpride does not interfere with blood sugar levels. Aripiprazole is also safe for diabetic patients.

47. E Serum lithium levels increase in the immediate postpartum period

Lithium is excreted in breast milk , so it should be explained clearly to the mother about the effect of lithium in newborn babies. Lithium can affect the baby during the second and third trimesters. It can have toxic effects if serum lithium levels are very high, and can also cause cardiac dysfunction, diabetes insipidus and hypothyroidism in the fetus. Lithium levels fall during the third trimester of pregnancy. However, immediately after delivery the serum concentration starts to rise, so lithium levels should be closely monitored. Lithium use is usually associated with Ebstein's anomaly of the tricuspid valve. Neural tube defects are seen with sodium valproate.

48. D Lithium

The rate of completed suicide in bipolar disorder is 15%. Meta-analysis by Baldessarini et al (2006) concluded that lithium reduced by 80% the risk of both attempted and completed suicides in patients with bipolar illness. Meta-analysis by Cipriani et al also has proved that lithium is superior to other mood stabilisers in all types of mood disorders.

49. D Grapefruit juice irreversibly blocks intestinal cytochrome P450

Several components in grapefruit, called furanocoumarins, irreversibly inhibit cytochrome P450 3A4 isoenzymes (CYP3A4) in the intestinal wall. Hence drugs that are metabolised (first-pass metabolism) in the intestinal wall by CYP3A4 enter the systemic circulation in increased quantities, leading to an increase in effects/side effects of the medication. One such example is grapefruit. Hence it is always advisable not to consume grapefruit juice when prescribed quetiapine.

50. B Convert sensitisation

This is an aversion conditioning using imagery. It is a form of therapy in which an undesirable behaviour is paired with an unpleasant image, in order to eliminate the behaviour. It is a form of sensitisation in which the conditioning process occurs in the imagination, out of sight (therefore covert rather than overt). It is useful in the treatment of alcoholism, smoking, chocolate addiction, nail tearing and overeating.

- **Aversion therapy:** the behaviour is modified by pairing undesirable behaviour with an unpleasant stimulus repeatedly.
- **Flooding:** the patient is in an undesired situation in vitro with the therapist for several hours until the original response diminishes.

- **Habituation:** through graded exposure from the least uncomfortable to the worst situation, for a period long enough for the undesired response to decline.
- **Implosion:** similar to flooding but the exposure to the undesired situation is imagined (in vivo).

51. E Reciprocal inhibition and systemic desensitisation

Reciprocal inhibition is defined as anxiety being inhibited by a feeling or response that is not compatible with the feeling of anxiety. Systematic desensitisation is also called graded exposure. It is used in the treatment of phobias. It involves teaching relaxation techniques to the patient and then a hierarchy of the fears is made so that the patient faces these fears from the least fearful situations to the most fearful, using relaxation techniques. The process of reciprocal inhibition paired with systematic desensitisation has proved effective in anxiety-related disorders.

52. A It is a process through which the child interprets new experiences by incorporating them into existing schema

According to Piaget's theory of cognitive development:

- Adaptation is a fundamental process that is made up of assimilation and accommodation.
- Assimilation is a process through which a child interprets new experiences by incorporating them into existing schema
- Accommodation is incorporating new experiences by modifying existing schema.
- Assimilation occurs before accommodation.

53. C 18–24 months

Piaget's theory of cognitive development explains about the different stages of cognitive development. According to this theory object permanence occurs during the sensorimotor stage. Object permanence is a child's ability to understand that, even if an object is not seen, heard or felt, it does exist. The research evidence indicates that it develops during the first 2 years although other researchers believe that it is a quality that is present by birth. However, there is no agreement about the onset of object permanence. Piaget believed that the child's understanding of the external world depended on motor development which linked tactile, visual and motor representations of the objects.

54. A Conservation

Piaget's theory of cognitive development explains the different stages of cognitive development. Conservation means a logical thinking, which refers to the child's ability to keep things the same irrespective of obvious changes. According to Piaget the ability of a child to understand that the amount or mass remains the same, even if it changes in shape, size or volume. It is the understanding that any quantity remains the same despite changes in the physical arrangement such as length or number, e.g. volume, a fat short glass holding 50 mL of liquid is the same as a tall thin glass holding 50 mL of liquid. Hypothetico-deductive reasoning is the ability to formulate a hypothesis and systematically test it to arrive at answers to questions posed at the verbal level.

55. E Transductive reasoning

Actions that are confined to exercising the innate reflexes are collectively called reflex activity. It occurs in the first stage of Piaget's theory.

56. D Non-logical thought is a feature of ages 7–11 years

The preoperational stage lasts from 2 years to 7 years, i.e. 5 years. Egocentric, non-logical thoughts and lack of conservation occur in the preoperational stage. Logical reasoning occurs in the concrete operational stage.

57. E Skinner

Skinner described operant conditioning which involves learning from one's environment. In classic conditioning, behaviour is developed or maintained mainly through reflexes or antecedents such as salivation while a dog hears a bell sound. Such behaviour is not maintained by the consequences. In operant conditioning, the behaviour is developed or maintained secondary to the consequences. Kohlberg is associated with the stages of moral development. Pavlov described classic conditioning. Piaget described the stages of cognitive development. Seligman described the concept of learned helplessness.

58. D Oral phase

According to Freud there are five stages of psychosexual development.

The approximate age range of the stages is characterised by:

- **Oral phase:** 1 year of fixation on mouth and lips – relation to sucking, biting and mouthing.
- **Anal phase:** 1–3 years of fixation on anal cavity – relation to toilet training.
- **Phallic phase:** 3–5/6 years of fixation and sensitivity to genitals. The Oedipus complex occurs only in this stage.
- **Latency phase:** 5/6 years of puberty – sexual preoccupations of earlier years repressed.
- **Genital phase:** puberty/maturity – new demands and sexual desires.

59. D Oedipus complex

This was described by Freud and occurs during the phallic stage of psychosexual development. See the explanation in the previous question for a description of the stages. The Oedipus complex derives its name from a classical Greek tragedy about Oedipus Rex who killed his father.

60. B 3 years

A 3-year-old child can copy a circle, show cooperative play, have imaginary companions and fear of animals, the dark and thunder, uses three- to four-word sentences and has a sexual identity.

A 4-year-old child can copy a cross and is toilet trained

At 4.5 years, a child can copy a square

At 5.5 years, a child can copy a triangle, use grammar in speech and play rule-governed games

At 7 years, a child can draw a diamond and has almost adult-like speech.

61. D Preoccupied/entangled

The adult attachment interview (AAI) is a semi-structured interview comprising 18 questions designed to assess the security of the adult's overall working model of attachment. It was developed by Mary Main. Based on the findings of AAI, four categories of adult attachment have been described:

- Secure/Autonomous: patients provide spontaneous, coherent answers in a non-defensive manner, whether the experiences are positive or negative.
- Dismissing: patients have avoidance patterns, give brief answers or provide a generalised positive description, but fail to provide evidence of these descriptions.
- Preoccupied: patients show multiple emotional responses with lengthy discussions of childhood memories and are often angry and tearful.
- Disorganised/unresolved: interrupted flow of thoughts makes the patient become incoherent and irrational.

There is an 80% correspondence between a mother's attachment category on AAI and her infant's attachment pattern on strange situation behaviour, developed by Mary Ainsworth.

62. C Assimilation

According to Piaget cognitive development has two concepts: cognitive structures and adaptation. Cognitive structures are understood in terms of schemas and operations. Schemas are basic building blocks of knowledge, organised patterns of thoughts and actions for understanding future experiences. Operations are mental actions that develop later in life. Adaptation is the process of adjustment and modifications to the demands of the environment. It is divided into assimilation and accommodation. In assimilation, new information is incorporated into already existing schemas without restructuring them. Accommodation is a complementary process in which the schema is modified to fit new experiences by restructuring the existing schemas. Equilibration is achieved when all information fits into schemas by either process of adaptation.

63. E Symbiosis

Mahler's developmental phases are:

- Normal autism (0–2 months): child's concerns centre on his or her own needs and child spends most of the time sleeping and eating.
- Symbiosis (2–5 months): a child perceives mother and self as one unit and separates it from the rest of the world.
- Differentiation (5–10 months): child starts differentiating self from mother
- Practising (10–18 months): increased interest in outer world and practises exploration.
- Rapprochement (18–24 months): becomes more autonomous, explores but requires reassurance on return.
- Object constancy (2–5 years): child understands that mother will not be lost if she is away temporarily and is able to explore outside world more independently.

64. E Moral reasoning in adults

Lawrence Kohlberg extended Piaget's theory. He studied moral reasoning in children, describing three major stages which included morality of preschool children (notion of avoiding punishment), conventional morality (notion of authority or mutual benefit) and principled morality (notion of generalised internalised moral principles).

65. D It leads to more aggression in patients undergoing catharsis

Catharsis is participation in activities such as running or kickboxing that allow a person to vent emotions, thereby reducing aggressive behaviour. Catharsis is thought to help some people discharge aggression whereas in others it may lead to more aggressive behaviours as a result of expressive behaviours.

66. D Preoperational

In the preoperational stage, children use a type of magical thinking, called phenomenalistic causality, in which events occurring together are thought to cause each other, e.g. thunder causes lightening and bad thoughts cause accidents. Children also use animistic thinking such as endowing feelings and intentions.

67. C Self-esteem

The self-concepts are how we see and think of ourselves. They include our self-esteem, which is how highly we rate ourselves, and our self-image, which is gained from other people's reactions towards us. The self-concept also includes your ideal self, which is how you would like to be seen.

Michael Argyle (2008) contended that there are four dimensions of the self:

1. **The self-image (perceived self):** this is the enduring aspects which vary with the different roles that we play. It contains a 'core' (sex, age, identity) and the roles played in a characteristic, individualised manner.
2. **Self-esteem:** this is how we judge ourselves compared with others. It is the value that we place in ourselves. Susan is clearly judging herself compared with her older sister.
3. **The ego-ideal:** this is the person whom we would ideally like to be and we usually aspire to become this person. Psychologists are interested in the gap between the perceived self (self-image) and the ideal self (ego-ideal).
4. **Integration of the self:** this is concerned with the consistency of the different elements of the self.

Ego-strength is not part of the four dimensions of the self.

68. D He passed the examination due to my hard work and academic prowess

Attribution error which takes into account the observed behaviour is called fundamental attribution error. It is the tendency to overvalue one's internal disposition such as personality, attributes, ability and motives of observed behaviour of other people, and at the same time undervalue external factors that may explain such behaviour. In other words, the person over-estimates the behaviour of others based on his or her observation of others. While explaining the behaviour of others a person neglects the effect of environmental factors influencing that behaviour. If a person is explaining his or her own behaviour they take into account the other factors that are influencing that behaviour.

69. E Reward

Five types of social powers were described by French and Raven. The power derived from the role is called authority. Coercive is power to punish and expert is power from skill, knowledge and experience. The power of reward is the ability to allocate resources and the power of referent is liked by others.

70. E Stereotyping of the victim of prejudice

The prejudice is a preconceived set of beliefs held about others which is not amenable to change. Discrimination is the enactment of prejudice. The prejudice could be reduced by providing equal status, cooperative effort and exposure to non-stereotypical individuals, and equality in the social environment.

71. B Awareness of the role of the interviewer

In delirium, the degree of impairment of orientation characteristically fluctuates. It is quite possible for the orientation to be intact at the particular time that the patient is being examined. Orientation includes awareness of time, place and person, i.e. interviewer.

72. B It is a good indicator of concentration

The serial sevens test is part of the MMSE. Although it has mathematical properties, it is primarily administered to test attention and concentration.

73. A It forms the basis of a therapy that aims to help people construct more effective interpretations and theories of the world

George Kelly (1905–1967) postulated personal-construct theory, in which he believed that we can engage in conscious mental activities and consequently know something about ourselves in the world. We can construct our lives or reconstruct the progress in our lives rather than just follow our impulses. We are able to identify invalid theories that hinder us and develop constructs in order to deal with all kinds of situations or events throughout our lives.

74. D Ready for action

Prochaska and DiClemente (1993) observed that patients came to see clinicians at different stages of readiness to make changes, and motivation was not a fixed and unchanging entity but fluctuated from day to day and in different circumstances. They saw these patients in different stages of motivation, including 'ready for action' when they will be willing to accept positive advice for change.

75. D Refer to social services

The initial management and measures to protect the child include a decision about separating the child from the family. There are particular difficulties in intervening in families where sexual abuse has occurred. These include a marked tendency to deny the seriousness of the abuse and of other family problems. If parents do not agree to separation, a care order can be made by the social services department.

76. B Fallacy of fairness

This means that the person judges a negative event as unfair when it isn't an issue of justice. Mental filtering means that the person picks out a single negative detail and dwells on it exclusively, while ignoring all the rest, so that all his or her reality becomes darkened. Reductionism means that the person fails to see the complex cause or the potential benefits of a situation. Instead, the person reduces it to a simple cause and a simple consequence. Emotional reasoning means that the person assumes that their negative emotions necessarily reflect the way things really are. Self-righteous cognitions mean that people should always do what they think is right and, if they don't, they are wrong and should be punished.

77. D Catastrophisation is a major mechanism

The cognitive theory of anxiety disorders suggests that the underlying danger-oriented beliefs predispose the individual to restrict attention to perceived threats in the environment. The individual makes catastrophic interpretations of ambiguous stimuli, underestimates his or her own coping resources and engages in dysfunctional 'safety behaviours' such as avoidance.

78. D Pre-evaluation

According to Prochaska and DiClemente (1993), patients come to clinicians at different stages of readiness to make changes in their behaviours and habits. Motivation is not a fixed or unchanging entity, but fluctuates from day to day and in different circumstances.

79. C These receptors are linked to sodium channels

Benzodiazepine receptors are associated with receptors for the inhibitory neurotransmitter γ-aminobutyric acid (GABA), which is linked to chloride channels. Zopiclone binds to the benzodiazepine receptor complex at a site that is different from that of benzodiazepines. Chlomethiazole binds to a site distinct from that of benzodiazepines and barbiturates. Zolpidem binds to a subtype of a binding site for benzodiazepine receptor-1, found on GABA neurons in the sensorimotor and extrapyramidal cortex.

80. D Serum lithium concentrations should be measured with changing renal function

Lithium is sensitive to the amount of water in the body. It is important to measure serum lithium concentrations, especially during electrolyte imbalances or changes in renal functioning, because there is a risk of toxicity that can prove to be life threatening. The target lithium concentration ranges between 0.4 and 0.8 mmol/L. Concentrations above 1 mmol/L are associated with an increased risk of toxicity. Lithium samples are taken 12 hours after the last dose.

81. B Diuretics alter the availability of lithium

Diuretics inhibit the renal excretion of lithium. It is important to alter the dose and monitor the serum concentration of lithium on initiation or alteration of the dose of diuretics. Sucralfate, which is used in the treatment of duodenal ulcer, reduces the absorption of amitriptyline by approximately 50%. Phenytoin is displaced from protein-binding sites by valproate. MAO inhibitors inhibit the metabolism of dietary amines and noradrenaline which they release, resulting in hypertension. Cytochrome P450 inhibits psychotropic metabolism.

82. C Failure of adequate trial occurs in 25% of patients

Almost 25% of patients fail to achieve an adequate trial with antidepressants. Antidepressants are effective in 65–70% of patients. Almost 50% of the partial responders to antidepressants benefit from the addition of lithium at a usual dose of 600–900 mg/day, with a treatment response observed in 2 weeks.

83. A 10–20% of patients show morphological kidney changes with long-term therapy

Approximately two-thirds (75%) of patients treated with lithium experience side effects. Of patients 10–20% demonstrate morphological changes in the kidney with long-term therapy. More than 1% of patients develop irreversible kidney failure after 10 years of treatment. The estimated risk of major congenital abnormalities for lithium-exposed babies is 4–12% compared with 2–4% in untreated controls. After 6–18 months of treatment, 5–35% of women develop subclinical or clinical hypothyroidism.

84. D Trazodone is a highly sedative tetracyclic antidepressant

Tetracyclic antidepressants such as maprotyline, mianserin and trazadone have marked sedating properties. Tetracyclic antidepressants have a sedative effect due to 5-hydroxytryptamine ($5HT_2$) and histamine antagonism. The least sedating tricyclic antidepressants are nortriptyline, protriptyline, and desipramine. The most sedating tricyclic antidepressants are amitriptyline, trimipramine, doxepin, imipramine and clomipramine. Tricyclic antidepressants have a sedative effect due to anticholinergic properties.

85. C Quetiapine

Reboxetine is a noradrenaline reuptake inhibitor that can cause side effects such as hypertension and hyponatraemia. Hence, regular blood pressure monitoring is required while on the medication. All the antidepressant medication has a risk of causing the side effect of hyponatraemia, although the propensity for mirtazapine may be slightly less. Quetiapine, although not an antidepressant, is licensed for augmentation in unipolar depression. Off-licence prescription may be appropriate but only with informed consent from the patient.

86. E An antipsychotic has not been prescribed

The National Institute for Health and Care Excellence (NICE) recommends that, for patients with bipolar disorder who have experienced chronic or recurrent depressive symptoms with functional impairment, while maintained on prophylactic medication, one can consider quetiapine where an antipsychotic has not been prescribed.

87. A Citalopram

Poststroke depression is a common problem seen in at least 30–40% of the survivors of intracerebral haemorrhage. There are significant risks associated with concurrent treatment of antidepressants with warfarin. Among the selective serotonin reuptake inhibitors (SSRIs), citalopram and sertraline appear to have the least interaction with warfarin. However, sertraline may be associated with a clinically non-significant increase in prothrombin time when used together with warfarin. Paroxetine can result in an increased bleeding tendency after several days of concurrent treatment with warfarin. Fluoxetine and fluvoxamine carry the highest risk of enhancing the effects of warfarin, and thereby increase bleeding potential. Dapoxetine, used in the treatment of premature ejaculation, was initially developed as a SSRI antidepressant. However, it has a rapid absorption and elimination rate, making it unsuitable as an antidepressant.

88. A Age of onset of psychosis is 2.7 years earlier in cannabis users

Large et al (2011) demonstrated that the age of onset of psychosis was 2.7 years earlier for those who abused cannabis regularly. The systematic meta-analysis also demonstrated a nil effect of alcohol on earlier presentation. For unidentified drug misuse the effect was about 2 years.

89. E Up to 80% of patients who experience a first episode psychosis relapse within 5 years of remission

Naturalistic long-term follow-up studies have shown that the early course of psychosis is characterised by repeated relapses. Up to 80% of first episode psychosis patients experience a relapse within a 5-year remission period from the initial episode.

90. A Boys experience more physical abuse than girls

Estimates of the prevalence of physical abuse vary with the criteria used. In the UK, about 3 young people per 1000 in the age range 0–18 years are on child protection registers. The most common forms of injuries are multiple bruising, burns, abrasions and bites, torn upper lips, bone fractures, subdural haemorrhage and retinal haemorrhage.

91. D Seeing vivid pictures in clouds

Sensory deception includes phenomena such as illusions and hallucinations. Seeing vivid images in clouds without any conscious effort is known as pareidolia, which is an illusion. All other options in the question are examples of sensory distortions, which are changes in perception as a result of a change in quality (e.g. xanthopsia; in derealisation, everything appears strange and unreal) and intensity (hyper- or hypoaesthesia, e.g. hyperacusis) of the stimulus or the spatial form (dysmegalopsia, e.g. metamorphopsia which means perceived irregularity in shape) of the perception.

92. A Dysmegalopsia

Pareidolia is vivid illusions without making any effort. They are the result of excessive fantasy thinking and vivid visual imagery. In hallucinosis, hallucinations occur in the absence of other psychotic features and include alcoholic hallucinosis and hallucinosis in Alzheimer's disease. Synaesthesia is the experience of a stimulus in one-sensory modality producing a sensory experience in another. It can occur under the influence of LSD (lysergic acid diethylamide). Phantom limb is an organic somatic hallucination of psychiatric origin. All of the above options are sensory deceptions whereas dysmegalospia (changes in spatial form) is a sensory distortion.

93. E Pareidolia is vivid illusions without any extra effort

Illusions are misinterpretations of stimuli arising from an external object. Illusions themselves are not indicative of any psychopathology, visual illusions being the most common ones. Pareidolia are vivid illusions without making any effort. They are the result of excessive fantasy thinking and vivid visual imagery. Affect illusions can be difficult to distinguish from hallucinations, e.g. a person with severe depression and delusion of guilt may say that other people are talking about killing him when in the company of others.

94. E Normal people can be persuaded to hallucinate

Hallucinations are not pathognomonic of any disorder. Normal people can also experience hallucinations. Similarly alcoholic hallucinosis is not a psychotic disorder. The Charles Bonnet syndrome is characterised by visual hallucination in people with impaired vision in clear consciousness. Lesions of the diencephalon can produce hallucinations, which are usually visual but can also be auditory. Alcoholic hallucinosis occurs in periods of relative abstinence after long-standing alcohol misuse.

95. D Reflex hallucination

This is a morbid form of synaesthesia. In it, a stimulus in one sensory field produces a hallucination in another. In functional hallucination, the stimulus is also experienced along with the hallucination, and the hallucination requires the presence of another real sensation. For example: 'I only hear the voices when water pipes are noisy.' Extracampine hallucinations are outside the limits of the sensory field. Sensory distortions are changes in perception that result from a change in quality and intensity of the stimulus or the spatial form of the perception.

96. C Characterised by akinetic mutism

Locked-in syndrome is a rare but specific condition characterised by akinetic mutism. There is full alertness and a feeling of aphonia, in which most of the muscles are paralysed except for blinking, eye movements and jaw movement. It is caused by a lesion in the motor pathways of the ventral pons. It is not a disorder of joints.

97. C Hysterical dissociation is present with apparent disorientation

Although established disorientation is indicative of an organic mental state, hysterical dissociation may present with apparent disorientation. Dissociative fugue may sometimes mimic disorientation. Therefore, disorientation makes a functional psychiatric disorder less likely but does not rule it out completely. Orientation in time is the first to be impaired followed by space and then by person. Loss of the knowledge of the patient's own name and identity comes last. Disorientation does not need clouding of consciousness, e.g. dementia.

98. A Memory of actual events is displaced in space and time

Confabulation is a falsification of memory in clear consciousness, in association with organically derived amnesia. It may include memories of actual events, which are displaced in time and space. The patient is usually not aware of memory deficits and hence a collateral history is essential to establish diagnosis. Autobiographical memory is most commonly affected. It is different from false memory syndrome, which is a much-debated concept in psychology; this means that normal individuals suddenly 'remember' supposedly repressed incidents of childhood abuse or other trauma. Confabulation may occur in Korsakoff's syndrome but it is not diagnostic of the condition. It can be easily confused with delusions and lying.

99. E Perseveration

A pathognomonic sign is decisively characteristic of a particular condition. Perseveration is probably the only pathognomonic sign in psychiatry. Other features mentioned in the question usually occur in organic brain disease but may also occur in functional psychiatric disorders.

100. B Cataplexy

This is collapse due to a sudden loss of muscle tone provoked by strong emotions such as hearing a bad news, crying and laughter. It is usually associated with narcolepsy. Catalepsy is characterised by perseveration of posture without any resistance to passive movements, and occurs in catatonia. Sleep paralysis can occur in healthy human beings or it may be present with narcolepsy, cataplexy and hallucinations while going to sleep.

101. C Primary delusion

Delusions can be classified as primary or secondary in nature depending on the underlying aetiology. Primary delusions occur independently of another psychopathological process such as a mood disorder. Secondary delusions are understandable in the given circumstances because of the pervasive mood or cultural content. Delusional misidentification syndromes include a number of discrete but related syndromes that have in common the concept of the double. Reflex hallucination is a morbid form of synaesthesia. In this, a stimulus in one sensory field produces a hallucination in another. Delusional percept is a type of primary delusion in which a normal perception is interpreted with a delusional meaning. The phenomenon described in the question is an example of a delusional percept.

102. E Pressure

Dimensions of delusional severity include extension, pressure, conviction, bizarreness, disorganisation, affective response and deviant behaviour. It is helpful to describe any delusion in these terms. Duration, content or frequency of delusional belief, and the diagnosis of mental disorder, do not suggest the severity of the delusion.

103. D Logoclonia

The repetition of syllables that occurs with parkinsonism is known as logoclonia. In echolalia, the patient repeats the words that are spoken to him without an understanding of their meaning. Echolalia is most often demonstrated in excited schizophrenia states, learning disability and organic states such as dementia. Echopraxia is when the patient imitates the interviewer's every action, despite the interviewer asking him not to. Automatic obedience is a condition in which the patient carries out every command in a literal and concrete fashion. Both echopraxia and automatic obedience are examples of excessive cooperation. Stuttering is not considered to be a psychopathological condition.

104. C Perseveration

This occurs when mental operations persist beyond the point of relevance. It is an example of perseveration; as in this case, whatever the question is the patient repeats the same answer, which is 'Monday'. His first answer has already served the purpose of the question and rest of the answers are senseless repetition. If a movement is carried out repeatedly, does not achieve any purpose or goal and is uniform, it is termed a 'stereotype'. Stuttering is not considered to be a psychopathological condition. Automatism implies that an action is taking place in the absence of consciousness. It usually occurs in epilepsy.

105. D It is a subjective experience

Depersonalisation is a subjective state of unreality. Ego-boundary disorders of schizophrenia are not classified as depersonalisation. Insight is preserved. Affect is always unpleasant. It can be found in temporal lobe disorders, hysterical dissociations and depressive illness. It could be impossible to make a distinction between depersonalisation and derealisation in some cases.

106. B Concentration

Attentional capacity is tested by the digit span task. In the MMSE, the serial sevens test assesses concentration. This test includes asking the patient to take 7 away from 100 and continue serially. Orientation is assessed for time, place and person. Executive functions are tested by frontal lobe tests such as Stroop's test and Luria's tests.

107. D Parapraxis

This is also called a freudian slip. It is an error in speech that is interpreted as occurring due to the interference of some unconscious ('repressed') wish, conflict or train of thought. The concept is thus part of classic psychoanalysis. Paragrammatism is a disorder of grammatical construction. Stock words are existing words that are used with individual symbolic meaning. Logoclonia is the repetition of syllables.

108. E Telegraphic speech

Broca's dysphasia is characterised by expressive aphasia. It includes difficulty in putting thoughts into words, and fluency is affected, words are omitted and sentences shortened. Less severe difficulty may look like telegramstyle speech. Conduction aphasia is a type of sensory or receptive aphasia. Scanning speech (e.g. in cerebellar lesions) and staccato speech (e.g. in multiple sclerosis) are examples of disorder of articulation (dysarthria). Fluent aphasia is receptive aphasia, which occurs in Wernicke's area lesions.

109. D *Mitgehen*

Mitmachen, *mitgehen*, echopraxia and *gegenhalten* are symptoms and signs of movement disorder. In echopraxia, an individual repeats another person's actions. If an individual moves his or her part of body in the direction of slight pressure it is called mitgehen, classified as an extreme form of cooperation. Gegenhalten is also called opposition in which an individual opposes all the movements that are passive with the same opposed degree of force.

110. A Déjà-vu

This is a feeling of familiarity in an unfamiliar situation. Jamais-vu is the opposite of déjà-vu. They can both occur as normal experiences or in temporal lobe epilepsy, cerebrovascular disorders and neurotic disorders. They are not primarily memory disorders. The other three options in the question are normal processes involved in the memory.

111. D Memory impairment due to electroconvulsive therapy includes apparent loss of memory stores

Electroconvulsive therapy (ECT) is most likely to impair memories of events immediately preceding the treatment, particularly more recent autobiographical memories. Memory impairment due to ECT includes impaired learning ability, defective retrieval and apparent loss of memory stores. In some cases, anterograde amnesia can also occur. In Korsakoff's syndrome, anterograde amnesia occurs due to problems at registration (encoding). Retrograde amnesia occurs after cerebral trauma due to impairment of retention (storage). Recognition is the retrieval of stored information which depends on the identification of items previously learned. Recall is the effortful retrieval of stored information. Confabulation is due to problems in retrieval. Registration can be impaired in fugue.

112. A Anger

According to the Kübler–Ross model of grief/coping with dying, there are five stages (acronym DABDA), such as denial, anger, bargaining, depression and acceptance. Not everyone goes through all the stages, and they do not necessarily follow a linear fashion. Some stages may be missed entirely, others may be experienced in a different order, some may be re-experienced repeatedly and some may get stuck in one of the stages. Mourning is the expression of bereavement.

113. D Overvalued idea

A person's idea of cleanliness is an acceptable and comprehensible idea but is pursued beyond the bounds of reason. Hence, it is termed an 'overvalued idea'. It is not a delusion because his belief is not morbid in origin. This belief is ego-syntonic and the person does not believe that it is 'senseless' so it is not an obsession. This person's concern for cleanliness is not an irrational fear of a specific situation so it is not a phobia.

114. C Mastery and control

This involves gaining a sense of control over a painful situation by confronting it directly and developing techniques that prevent feelings of being overwhelmed. Humour involves counteracting painful affects by seeing the comic side of a humour situation. Sublimation involves using past-traumatic or unpleasant experiences, emotions as well as basic 'id drives' in a way that both reduces anxiety and is not injurious to society. Denial and reaction formation are neurotic/immature ego-defence mechanisms.

115. A Countertransference

The term 'countertransference' is used in a number of different ways by psychodynamic therapists. It most commonly refers to the therapist's emotional response to the patient. The therapist's response will be made up of his or her own 'transference' feelings which have a basis in the therapist's own prior experiences and the therapist's reaction to patient's transference towards him or her.

116. B Eugen Bleuler

It was Bleuler who replaced the term 'dementia praecox' by 'schizophrenia'. Kraepelin coined the term 'dementia praecox'. Morel coined the term *'démence précoce'*. Kahlbaum coined the term 'catatonia'. Kraepelin distinguished between manic depression and dementia praecox, which was later named schizophrenia. Adolf Meyer was the founder of psychobiology.

117. D Kraepelin

He translated the term *'démence précoce'* into dementia praecox.

118. E Morel

Benedict Morel (1809–1873) was a French psychiatrist. He had used the term *'démence précoce'* to describe the group of patient who had deteriorated mental illness with an onset in adolescence.

119. C Cultural bias in testing of IQ

Raven's Progressive Matrices were devised to overcome cultural biases and they contain a number of non-verbal pattern matching exercises. Although we know that the art of pattern matching is used more in some cultures than others, it can still be culturally influenced.

120. A Emotions

Plutchik, in 1980, suggested eight primary emotions, which are in four pairs of opposites represented in Plutchik's wheel. Intelligence, which is measured as intelligence quotient (IQ), refers to mental age divided by chronological age multiplied by 100. Personality theories have mainly two groups, namely idiographic (based on a person's unique characteristics) and nomothetic (based on dimensions and traits common to all). Perception includes gestalt principles (Rubin Vase). Memory is composed of registration, storage and retrieval.

121. E Winnicott

Winnicott believed that mothers supply a holding environment in which infants are contained and experienced. The mother needs to be 'good-enough' but not perfect, to bring the world to the child and offer empathy for the infant's needs. If the mother is attentive to her baby's needs the infant can become more attuned to his or her own bodily functions and drives; this forms the basis for a gradually evolving sense of self.

122. A Dream work is the process by which unconscious wishes are processed into dreams

Secondary revision refers to the ego organising the primitive aspects of dreams to a more coherent form. Freud stated that dreams are manifestations of unconscious childhood wishes. The manifest content is what the dreamer recalls and the latent content is the unconscious thoughts and wishes in the dreams.

123. E Using the term 'démence précoce'

Ewold Hacker described bizarre symptoms in hebephrenia. Kretschmer described schizophrenia in people with an 'asthenic' body type. Langfeldt described 'true schizophrenia'. Kraepelin differentiated patients with schizophrenia and manic–depressive psychosis.

124. A Catatonic symptoms are frequently found among patients in developing countries

The international pilot study of schizophrenia showed that it was possible to conduct assessments across cultures using standardised diagnostic instruments and that the core symptoms of schizophrenia showed little variation. It also showed that catatonic symptoms were more common in developing countries. The follow-up study found that at 2-year follow-up patients in the developing countries fared better.

125. E The incidence of mania is the same in ethnic minorities living in developed countries as that of the native population

The broad diagnosis of schizophrenia (lacking schneiderian symptoms) showed a three-fold difference across countries. Studies have shown that a broad diagnosis of schizophrenia has increased incidence, reflecting the role of psychosocial factors. At 2 years, patients in developing countries were better despite the increased incidence of acute-onset illness. Mania is seen to increase in ethnic minorities. African and Caribbean countries experience more psychosis in mania.

126. D Infant is exposed to escalating amounts of stress

Ainsworth developed the strange situation to assess the quality and security of an infant's attachment. In this test, the infant is exposed to escalating amounts of stress. The protocol has seven steps. According to Ainsworth's studies, about 65% of infants are securely attached by the age of 24 months.

Chapter 4

Test questions: 4

Questions: MCQs

For each question, select one answer option.

HISTORY AND MENTAL STATE EXAMINATION

1. Which of the following factors is desirable when conducting a psychiatric interview?

    A   Closed questions allow free exchange of information
    B   Only factual information provided by the patient is considered
    C   Open questions are preferred at the end of the interview if time permits
    D   Polythematic questions save time
    E   Recapitulation of information is encouraged

2. A 76-year-old man presented at the outpatient clinic with memory problems. He had difficulty expressing himself and complained of low mood, being forgetful and difficulties with activities of daily living, e.g. shopping. He was well until 18 months ago when he woke up with a limp that has persisted ever since then. What is the most likely diagnosis?

    A   Alzheimer's disease
    B   Delirium
    C   Dementia with Lewy bodies
    D   Severe depression
    E   Vascular dementia

3. During a Mental State Examination, a 23-year-old male patient included irrelevant details before coming to the point. Which of the following best describes this?

    A   Circumstantiality
    B   Clang association
    C   Flight of ideas
    D   Neologism
    E   Tangentiality

4. An 18-year-old woman presented to the accident and emergency department with dehydration, low mood and binge eating. The on-call psychiatrist observed calluses on her knuckles. Which of the following signs is associated with the above disorder?

    A   Kayser–Flescher ring
    B   Lanugo hair
    C   Osler's nodes
    D   Russell's sign
    E   Xanthelasma

5. The clinician asked a patient 'What has brought you to the hospital today?'. What type of questioning style is being used?

  A   Closed question
  B   Compound question
  C   Directive question
  D   Leading question
  E   Open question

6. A psychiatric trainee asks too many question in an interview such as 'Do you feel low, hopeless and helpless about future?'. Which questioning style is being used in the psychiatric interview?

  A   Closed question
  B   Compound question
  C   Directive question
  D   Leading question
  E   Open question

7. What is the phenomenon in which thoughts are associated by the sound of words rather than by their meaning called?

  A   Circumstantiality
  B   Clang association
  C   Flight of ideas
  D   Neologism
  E   Tangentiality

COGNITIVE ASSESSMENT

8. The Mini-Mental State Examination (MMSE) is a commonly used battery in the assessment of cognitive functioning. Which of the following statements about MMSE is correct?

  A   It does not assess frontal lobe functioning
  B   It is a 26-point scale
  C   It is the best diagnostic tool for Alzheimer's disease
  D   It is a culture-free test
  E   It is a self-rated scale

9. Which of the following is a commonly used test to detect prefrontal dysfunction?

  A   Benton's visual retention test
  B   Digit-span task
  C   Raven's progressive matrices
  D   Rey–Osterrieth complex figure test
  E   Wisconsin card sorting test

10. Which of the following tests is used to detect impairment of everyday memory function and determine the effects of disease progression?

  A   Auditory verbal learning test
  B   California verbal learning test
  C   Digit-span task
  D   Rivermead behavioural memory test
  E   Wechsler memory scale III

11. Which of the following statements about Brewin's dual representational model of post-traumatic stress disorder is correct?

    A   A considerable amount of traumatic experience-related information is stored as situationally accessible memory

    B   Situationally accessible memory can be edited and incorporated into a person's autobiographical memory

    C   Situationally accessible memory can be retrieved deliberately

    D   Situationally accessible memory is dependent on the hippocampus

    E   Verbally accessible memory is dependent on the amygdala

12. Which of the following syndromes is a 'mirror image' of prosopagnosia?

    A   Capgras' syndrome

    B   Charles Bonnet syndrome

    C   Cotard's syndrome

    D   Diogenes syndrome

    E   Fregoli's syndrome

13. Which of the following tests measures a patient's premorbid level of intelligence?

    A   Cambridge cognitive examination

    B   Wechsler test of adult reading

    C   Wechsler abbreviated scale of intelligence

    D   Wechsler adult intelligence scale

    E   Wechsler intelligence scale for children

14. Which of the following is a test of executive functions?

    A   Doors and people test

    B   Rey auditory verbal learning test

    C   Rey–Osterrieth test

    D   Rivermead behavioural memory test

    E   Wisconsin card sorting test

15. You are assessing intelligence (or IQ) of a 15-year-old boy who is from south Asia. He cannot speak, read or write in English. Which of the following IQ tests will be most suitable in this situation?

    A   Bender gestalt test

    B   Raven's progressive matrices

    C   Stanford–Binet test

    D   Wechsler adult intelligence scale III

    E   Wechsler intelligence scale for children

16. A 70-year-old man presents with memory problems. He has completed schooling with two general certificates of secondary education and worked as a painter most of his life. What is the minimum score that he should have on the MMSE to raise the possibility of dementia?

    A   22 or less

    B   23 or less

    C   24 or less

    D   25 or less

    E   26 or less

17. Which of the following conditions results in retrograde memory loss?

    A   Acute closed head injury
    B   Diencephalic amnesia
    C   Hippocampal amnesia
    D   Transient epileptic amnesia
    E   Transient global amnesia

NEUROLOGICAL EXAMINATION

18. A 39-year-man with alcohol dependence told you that he went out drinking and then fell asleep in the kitchen on returning to his apartment. He could no longer grip firmly with his right hand. Which of the following signs will you find on examination?

    A   Claw hand
    B   Decreased sensation over the little finger and half the ring finger
    C   Paralysis of the thenar muscles
    D   Wasting of the interossei muscles
    E   Wrist drop

19. A 46-year-old woman presents with complaints of a sudden onset of pain in the lower back and right thigh, which radiates down into the leg. You think that the patient has an L5–S1 disc prolapse. Which of the following findings would not be consistent with this provisional diagnosis?

    A   Calf pain
    B   Increased ankle jerk
    C   Increased sensation on the outer dorsum of the foot
    D   Weak foot plantar extension
    E   Weak knee extension

20. A 30-year-old woman mentioned that she has been trying to conceive without success. She has amenorrhoea for some time and at times has noticed a milky discharge from her breasts. On neurological examination, which of the following signs is likely to be noticed?

    A   Absolute central scotoma
    B   Bitemporal hemianopia
    C   Centrocaecal scotoma
    D   Inferior quadrantic homonymous hemianopia
    E   Superior quadrantic homonymous hemianopia

21. Your consultant informed you that a 33-year-old man has a lateral medullary syndrome. He asked, 'What signs you would expect to see on clinical examination?'.

    A   Contralateral ataxia
    B   Contralateral homonymous hemianopia
    C   Contralateral Horner's syndrome
    D   Crossed pattern sensory loss
    E   Ptosis

22. A 53-year-old man presents with a left -sided weakness. On neurological examination, he has left hemiplegia, left hemisensory loss of face and arm, and left neglect. What is the most likely cause?

    A   Left anterior cerebral artery occlusion
    B   Left middle cerebral artery occlusion
    C   Posterior cerebral artery occlusion
    D   Right anterior cerebral artery occlusion
    E   Right middle cerebral artery occlusion

ASSESSMENT

23. A 79-year-old man presented with 1-year history of cognitive decline, particularly with impairment in attention and visuospatial ability, visual hallucinations and vivid dreams. Which is the most likely diagnosis?

    A   Alzheimer's disease
    B   Delirium tremens
    C   Dementia of Lewy bodies
    D   Normal pressure hydrocephalus
    E   Vascular dementia

24. A 38-year-old married woman has a 10-year history of nausea, abdominal pain, skin blotchiness and dysmenorrhoea. The symptoms have been extensively investigated but no cause has been identified. What is the most likely diagnosis?

    A   Body dysmorphic disorder
    B   Hypochondriasis
    C   Malingering
    D   Neurasthenia
    E   Somatisation disorder

25. A 33-year-old single man presented at the emergency department. He had a naloxone eyedrop test while he was treated at another hospital. On what was he dependent?

    A   Alcohol
    B   Amphetamines
    C   Benzodiazepines
    D   Opioids
    E   Zopiclone

26. Two students took a set of examinations. One of them who had practised questions from the previous year's examinations got a better score than the other, who read textbooks and had a wider knowledge of the subject. Which of the following is most likely to have occurred?

    A   Barnum effect
    B   Halo effect
    C   Hawthorne effect
    D   Practice effect
    E   Recency effect

27. Which of the following is the most appropriate assessment tool for measuring the severity and change in psychotic symptoms?

    A   Brief psychiatric rating scale
    B   General health questionnaire
    C   Neuropsychiatric inventory
    D   Present state examination
    E   Schedules for clinical examination in psychiatry

28. Which of the following brain imaging scans would best help distinguish Alzheimer's disease from dementia of Lewy bodies?

    A   CT scan
    B   DAT scan
    C   Functional MRI
    D   Perfusion SPECT
    E   Structural MRI

29. One month after the death of her husband, a 64-year-old woman visited her general practitioner. She was pining for her husband and was still very tearful. She had poor sleep, poor appetite, felt comforted by the voice of her late husband and felt his presence late at night. What is the most likely diagnosis?

    A   Adjustment disorder
    B   Depression
    C   Stage 1 of grief reaction
    D   Stage 2 of grief reaction
    E   Stage 3 of grief reaction

AETIOLOGY

30. A 20-year-old single man presented with mood incongruent complex delusions and social withdrawal over the past 1 year. Which of the following risk factors would have contributed to his illness?

    A   Drinking 80 units of alcohol per week
    B   Human leukocyte antigen (HLA)-B27 factor in blood
    C   Loss of mother before age 11 years
    D   Migrated from another country
    E   Wearing hearing aid for loss of hearing

31. Which of the following is associated with the risk of being violent as a child?

    A   Attention deficit hyperactivity disorder
    B   Autistic spectrum disorder
    C   Cocaine use in pregnancy
    D   Mother in prison
    E   Youngest child of family

32. According to family studies of panic disorders, what is the age-adjusted risk to the first-degree relatives of probands with panic disorder?

    A   0–1 times higher
    B   2–4 times higher
    C   4–8 times higher
    D   6–8 times higher
    E   8–10 times higher

33. Which maternal vitamin is most likely to be associated with an increased risk of developing schizophrenia in the child?

    A   Vitamin A
    B   Vitamin B_1
    C   Vitamin C
    D   Vitamin D
    E   Vitamin E

34. Kendler's twin studies showed an increased association between life events and the number of previous depressive episodes leading to a new depressive episode. What is the association between stressful life events and depressive episodes in patients with a family history of depression?

A   Decreases
B   Increases
C   Inversely related
D   Not associated
E   Remains the same

35. According to Andreasson et al (1987), what is the probable cause of schizophrenia?

A   Birth anomalies
B   Brain structure
C   Environmental cause
D   Genetics
E   Neurodevelopmental

36. What is the likely 'season of birth effect' for patients with schizophrenia?

A   April, May, June
B   January, February, March
C   July, August
D   November, December
E   September, October

37. A chronic feeling of self-defeat increases the risk of developing certain mental disorders. Which of the following is the most likely mental disorder?

A   Anxiety
B   Depression
C   Mania
D   Obsessive–compulsive disorder
E   Schizophrenia

DIAGNOSIS

38. A 29-year-old single man presents with odd forms of communication, ideas of reference, illusions, suspiciousness and poor rapport with others. He also described obsessive ruminations without inner resistance and unusual perceptual experiences. What is the most likely diagnosis?

A   Anankastic personality disorder
B   Histrionic personality disorder
C   Paranoid personality disorder
D   Schizoid personality disorder
E   Schizotypal personality disorder

39. A 19-year old male university student presents with a 6-month history of social withdrawal, hearing voices and believing that he had a special mission to stop terrorism in the whole world. He denied any history of drug abuse. What is the most likely diagnosis?

A   Acute polymorphic psychotic disorder
B   Delirium tremens
C   Manic episode
D   Persistent delusional disorder
E   Schizophrenia

40. A 17-year-old man presents with low mood, cognitive disturbances and recurrent repetitive thoughts of hurting people. He has had the symptoms for 3 months without an obvious trigger. What is the most likely diagnosis?

   A   Asperger's syndrome
   B   Depressive episode.
   C   Obsessive–compulsive disorder
   D   Prodromal symptoms of psychotic disorder
   E   Schizophrenia

41. A 30-year-old man has excessive perspiration when exposed to feared situations. He avoids small group gatherings due to fear of humiliation, and at times has fleeting thoughts of suicide. What is the most likely diagnosis?

   A   Agoraphobia
   B   Dependent personality disorder
   C   Depressive episode
   D   Generalised anxiety disorder
   E   Social phobia

CLASSIFICATION

42. Which of the following is included under schizophrenia in the *International Classification of Disease*, 10th revision (ICD-10)?

   A   Disorganised schizophrenia
   B   Post-schizophrenic depression
   C   Schizoaffective disorder
   D   Schizophreniform disorder
   E   Schizotypal disorder

43. When was the fourth edition of the *Diagnostic and Statistical Manual of Mental Disorders* (DSM-IV) published?

   A   1954
   B   1964
   C   1974
   D   1984
   E   1994

44. According to the DSM-IV, which axis does autistic disorder belong to?

   A   Axis I
   B   Axis II
   C   Axis III
   D   Axis IV
   E   Axis V

45. Which of the following is categorised as a personality disorder according to the DSM-IV?

   A   Anankastic personality disorder
   B   Anxious personality disorder
   C   Dissocial personality disorder
   D   Histrionic personality disorder
   E   Narcissistic personality disorder

46. A 32-year-old man was diagnosed with a persistent delusional disorder. What is the minimum duration of symptoms required to qualify for an ICD-10 diagnosis?

- A   2 weeks
- B   1 month
- C   3 months
- D   6 months
- E   24 months

47. In which of the following categories of the ICD-10 is neurasthenia classified?

- A   Dissociative (conversion) disorder
- B   Other anxiety disorder
- C   Other neurotic disorder
- D   Reaction to severe stress and adjustment disorder
- E   Somatoform disorder

48. Which of the following categories of the ICD-10 includes factitious disorder?

- A   Dissociative (conversion) disorder
- B   Enduring personality changes, not attributable to brain damage and disease
- C   Mixed and other personality disorder
- D   Other disorders of adult personality and behaviour
- E   Specific personality disorders

49. Which of the following statements is not part of the diagnostic criteria for emotionally unstable personality disorder in the ICD-10?

- A   Chronic feeling of emptiness
- B   Involvement in intense and unstable relationships
- C   Recurrent threats or acts of self-harm
- D   Transient stress-related paranoid ideation
- E   Uncertainty about self-image

50. What is the minimum duration of symptoms required to meet the diagnostic criteria for cyclothymia in the ICD-10?

- A   1 month
- B   4 months
- C   6 months
- D   12 months
- E   24 months

BASIC PSYCHOPHARMACOLOGY

51. Which of the following is the most suitable antipsychotic drug supported by available data in respect of its effectiveness in the treatment of the negative symptoms of schizophrenia?

- A   Amisulpride
- B   Flupenthixol
- C   Olanzapine
- D   Risperidone
- E   Zuclopenthixol

52. Adverse sexual effects are common with antidepressant therapy. Which of the following is a correct match for the approximate prevalence of this side effect with an antidepressant drug?

    A   10% with trazodone
    B   40% in monoamine oxidase inhibitors
    C   60% in tricyclic antidepressants
    D   60–70% with selective serotonin reuptake inhibitors
    E   80% in venlafaxine

53. Hypersomnia/sedation was found to be the most common side effect in clinical antipsychotic trials of the effectiveness of intervention. Which drug is an exception to these findings?

    A   Olanzapine
    B   Perphenazine
    C   Quetiapine
    D   Risperidone
    E   Ziprasidone

54. A 24-year-old man has undergone heroin detoxification on the ward. He does not want an opioid maintenance therapy. He has requested medication that could help him to maintain abstinence. What is the drug of choice?

    A   Codeine
    B   Disulfiram
    C   Lofexidine
    D   Naloxone
    E   Naltrexone

55. Which of the following statements about naltrexone is correct?

    A   In opiate-dependent patients, naltrexone therapy reduces the risk of suicide
    B   Naltrexone acts on all three types of opioid receptors
    C   Naltrexone causes a fall in blood pressure in opiate-dependent individuals
    D   Naltrexone is an opioid agonist
    E   Naltrexone is short acting

56. What is the mechanism of action of acamprosate?

    A   5-Hydroxytryptamine (5-HT_2) antagonism
    B D_2-receptor antagonism
    C γ-Aminobutyric acid A (GABA-A) antagonism
    D   GABA transaminase inhibitor
    E N-Methyl-D-aspartate receptor antagonism

57. Clozapine causes hypersalivation in some patients. What is the most likely mechanism of action?

    A 5-HT_2 antagonism
    B α_1-Receptor antagonism
    C α_2-Receptor antagonism
    D D_1-Receptor antagonism
    E   Muscarinic receptor antagonism

58. Which of the following 5-hydroxytryptamine (5-HT) receptors is ligand gated ion channel receptor?

    A 5-HT_1
    B 5-HT_2
    C 5-HT_3
    D 5-HT_4
    E 5-HT_5

59. Which of the following drugs acts as competitive antagonist in the 5-HT$_3$ receptors?

A   Clozapine
B   Flupenthixol
C   Fluphenazine
D   Haloperidol
E   Risperidone

60. A 45-year-old man with alcohol dependence has been prescribed Antabuse for the past 2 months. He stopped taking it 3 days ago. He has consumed a glass of lager today and developed severe hypotension, flushing, sweating and sickness. What is the most likely reason behind this?

A   Antabuse irreversibly blocks aldehyde dehydrogenase
B   Antabuse is still in his system
C   Antabuse sensitises a person to alcohol
D   His drink might have been spiked
E   His physical symptoms are unrelated to Antabuse use

61. A 34-year-old man presented to you with involuntary movements and cirrhosis of the liver. On examination, he was found to have a ring in his cornea. What is the most likely diagnosis?

A   Alcohol dependence
B   Chronic antipsychotic therapy
C   Huntington's disease
D   Hypercholesterolemia
E   Wilson's disease

62. D-Penicillamine is used in patients with Wilson's disease. What is the mechanism of action of D-penicillamine?

A   Agonism
B   Chemical antagonism
C   Irreversible competitive antagonism
D   Non-competitive antagonism
E   Reversible competitive antagonism

63. What is the elimination half-life of lithium?

A   5 hours
B   10 hours
C   15 hours
D   20 hours
E   40 hours

64. Which of the following drugs is excreted unchanged from the body?

A   Amisulpride
B   Carbamazepine
C   Lithium
D   Olanzapine
E   Risperidone

65. Which of the following is an acute side effect of lithium therapy?

A   Hair loss
B   Hypothyroidism
C   Kidney damage
D   Peripheral neuropathy
E   Tremor

BASIC PSYCHOLOGICAL PROCESSES

66. A 7-year-old boy was scared when his family got a new cat in their home. When in the same room as the cat, the boy stayed calm provided that he could sit with his mother and receive his favourite chocolate. Which of the following is the most likely theoretical principle?

    A   Aversive conditioning
    B   Avoidance learning
    C   Classic conditioning
    D   Operant conditioning
    E   Reciprocal inhibition

67. Pairing of an unpleasant stimulus with the target behaviour is seen in the use of Antabuse when associated with alcohol dependence to maintain abstinence. Which is the most likely phenomenon?

    A   Aversive conditioning
    B   Avoidance learning
    C   Extinction
    D   Operant conditioning
    E   Reciprocal inhibition

68. A 15-year-old boy received painkiller injections from his general practitioner every day to treat back pain. Initially, he had panic attacks every time, just before he received the injection. He has now started experiencing panic attacks while in the waiting area in the clinic. What is the most likely phenomenon?

    A   Avoidance
    B   Classic conditioning
    C   Flooding
    D   Operant conditioning
    E   Reciprocal inhibition

69. The above boy continued to attend the clinic for follow-ups but no longer received painkilling injections. After 3 months, he no longer had panic attacks. What is the most likely phenomenon?

    A   Avoidance
    B   Extinction
    C   Flooding
    D   Implosion
    E   Punishment

BASIC PSYCHOLOGY

70. A 40-year-old man believed that he was having a heart attack after feeling breathless. What is the most likely phenomenon?

    A   All-or-none thinking
    B   Black-and-white thinking
    C   Catastrophic thinking
    D   Minimisation
    E   Selective abstraction

71. A 29-year-old male trainee accountant passed the first 2 years of examinations but failed the last year. Since failing, he had started to think that he was 'good for nothing'. Which is the most likely cognitive bias?

    A   Arbitrary inference
    B   Catastrophic thinking
    C   Dichotomous thinking
    D   Overgeneralisation
    E   Personalisation

72. A 75-year-old man died as a result of a cardiac arrest in the intensive care unit. The treating doctor believed that he was responsible for the patient's death despite knowing that the patient had a poor prognosis. Which is the most likely cognitive distortion?

    A   Arbitrary inference
    B   Catastrophic thinking
    C   Dichotomous thinking
    D   Overgeneralisation
    E   Personalisation

73. A 21-year-old woman saw her boyfriend talking to another girl on the telephone and started thinking that her boyfriend was cheating on her. Which is the most likely cognitive distortion?

    A   Arbitrary inference
    B   Catastrophisation
    C   Dichotomous thinking
    D   Overgeneralisation
    E   Personalisation

HUMAN PSYCHOLOGICAL DEVELOPMENT

74. At what age do colour vision and accommodation develop?

    A   1 month
    B   2 months
    C   4 months
    D   6 months
    E   Birth

75. A 4-year-old boy experimented with 'eating by himself with confidence'. What stage of Erickson's psychosocial development is represented in this case?

    A   Autonomy versus shame
    B   Industry versus inferiority
    C   Initiative versus guilt
    D   Intimacy versus isolation
    E   Trust versus mistrust

76. Which of the following Kohlberg's stages is correctly matched with age?

    A   Conventional: 13–16 years
    B   Preconventional: birth to 2 years
    C   Preconventional: 2–7 years
    D   Postconventional: 12–16 years
    E   Postconventional: 13–16 years

77. Which of the following statements about the assessment of attachment is correct?

   A   Attachment is decreased by anxiety
   B   Attachment is increased if the mother is hostile towards her child
   C   Attachment theory was developed by Thomas and Chess
   D   Father cannot be a primary caregiver
   E   The need for food tends to motivate attachment more than need for closeness

78. Which of the following statements is consistent with the concept of imprinting?

   A   It is a concept used by psychiatrists to understand the effects of group living on child development
   B   It is associated with Martin Seligman
   C   It was described by Nikolas Tinbergen successfully in eliciting specific behaviour
   D   Lorenz described newly hatched goslings programmed to follow a movable object
   E   The term 'imprinting' was coined by Karl Von Frish

79. Which of the following describes the 'choo-choo' phenomenon correctly?

   A   It consists of children's words for a steam engine locomotive
   B   It forms the basis of all animal behaviours
   C   It refers to an effect of social isolation in early life
   D   It is an encouragement to explore and engage in a lot of play acts
   E   It is the actual psychological alignment in peer-only-reared infant monkeys

80. Which of the following statements is consistent with human aggressive behaviour?

   A   It always implies intent to harm or injure another person
   B   It assumes the form of non-violent actions
   C   It refers to mainly physical attacks against oneself
   D   It increases when the onset of the mental disorder is acute
   E   It involves familiar person generalisation with the exception of male adolescents

81. Which of the following statements is consistent with the concept of extinction?

   A   It is associated with Charles Darwin
   B   It completely destroys a conditioned response
   C   It is a condition in which a conditioned stimulus is transferred from one stimulus to another
   D   It is where the conditioned stimulus is constantly repeated without the unconditioned stimulus
   E   It follows partial recovery

82. Who developed the theory of learning known as operant conditioning?

   A   Albert Bandura
   B   BF Skinner
   C   EL Thorndike
   D   Ivan Pavlov
   E   JB Watson

SOCIAL PSYCHOLOGY

83. At work, a 30-year-old man was constantly made fun of for being the only homosexual man there. Which stage of Allport's scale of prejudice and discrimination best describes the above scenario?

   A   Antilocution

B   Attack
C   Avoidance
D   Discrimination
E   Instrumental aggression

84. As a small businessman, a 37-year-old man voted for the political party that cut taxes and spent less on welfare. According to Katz (1960), which function of the attitude does the above best describe?

A   Accuracy function
B   Ego-defensive function
C   Instrumental function
D   Knowledge function
E   Value-expressive function

DESCRIPTION AND MEASUREMENT

85. Which of the following rating scales can be used reliably for psychometric assessment of personality?

A   California personality inventory
B   General health questionnaire
C   Montgomery–Åsberg depression rating scale
D   Present state examination
E   Symptoms sign inventory

86. Which of the following statements about the reliability of the diagnosis of mental disorders is correct?

A   It is generally high because the criteria are polythetic
B   It is high for histrionic personality disorder
C   It is high for schizophrenia diagnosed by Bleuler's criteria
D   It is low for antisocial personality disorder
E   It improves along with validity by using operational criteria

BASIC PSYCHOLOGICAL TREATMENTS

87. Which of the following is central to the schema therapy?

A   Appreciation of patient's understanding of 'theory of mind'
B   Consideration of subconscious defence mechanisms
C   Detailed exploration of reciprocal roles
D   Targeting of emotional regulation and distress tolerance
E   Understanding of the origin and adoption of unhelpful 'modes'

88. Which of the following concepts is associated with dialectic behaviour therapy formulation?

A   Catharsis
B   Paradoxical gain
C   Primary gain
D   Radical acceptance
E   Secondary gain

89. Which of the following principles applies to motivational interviewing?

    A   Avoiding discrepancy
    B   Confrontation
    C   Reciprocal roles
    D   Rolling with resistance
    E   Schemas

90. Which of the following psychological therapies uses hypothesising and circular questioning?

    A   Cognitive–analytical therapy
    B   Dialectic behaviour therapy
    C   Flooding
    D   Systematic desensitisation
    E   Systemic family therapy

91. Which of the following psychological treatments uses sequential diagrammatic reformulation?

    A   Abreaction
    B   Catharsis
    C   Cognitive-analytic therapy
    D   Cognitive-behavioural therapy
    E   Ventilation

PREVENTION OF PSYCHIATRIC DISORDER

92. Which of the following statements about prevention is correct?

    A   Continuation of mood stabilisers in patients with bipolar affective disorder is a type of primary prevention
    B   Educating pregnant women about the hazards of substance misuse is a type of secondary prevention
    C   Educating teenagers about the hazards of alcohol misuse is a type of secondary prevention
    D   Preventive measures in alcohol misuse are more effective when focused on the heavy drinkers than on the general population
    E   Random screening of drivers for breath alcohol levels is a form of primary prevention

93. According to current research evidence, which of the following has been found to be ineffective in the prevention of a relapse of recurrence in patients with bipolar affective disorder?

    A   Carbamazepine
    B   Chlorpromazine
    C   Haloperidol
    D   Lithium
    E   Topiramate

94. Which of the following is a primary preventive strategy for alcohol misuse?

    A   Facilitating early recognition of hazardous drinking by questionnaires
    B   Fostering moderate informal drinking and promoting awareness of hazards
    C   Involvement of Alcoholics Anonymous
    D   Prescription of disulfiram
    E   Total abstinence

95. Which of the following drugs is associated with fetal Epstein's anomaly?

A   Chlorpromazine
B   Haloperidol
C   Lamotrigine
D   Lithium
E   Sodium valproate

DESCRIPTIVE PSYCHOPATHOLOGY

96. Which of the following statements about depersonalisation is correct?

A   It is associated with altered consciousness
B   It is associated with an unpleasant emotional state
C   It is absent in normal people
D   People around them feel unreal
E   Perception of time is not altered

97. Which of the following statements about learned helplessness is correct?

A   In learned helplessness, punishment is contingent upon the action
B   It has been demonstrated in animal experiments
C   It is an example of classic conditioning
D   It results in the ability to escape from stressful situations
E   The theory of learned helplessness was first contested by Skinner

98. Which of the following statements is consistent with pseudo-hallucinations?

A   They are not part of normal experience
B   They are associated with flat affect
C   They occur in Ganser's syndrome
D   They tend to occur mainly in visual modality
E   They indicate the presence of psychosis

99. Which of the following distinguishes mania from hypomania?

A   Elevated mood
B   Increased energy
C   Irritability
D   Pressure of speech
E   Severe interference with social functioning

100. 'There is no hiding place for me in this world. They always keep an eye on me day and night. I hear a male voice reporting me to his boss about my movements.' What does this phenomenon represent?

A   Delusion of control
B   Delusion of persecution
C   Delusion of reference
D   Running commentary
E   Thought insertion

101. 'My family often knows that I don't trust them, even without me telling them and even when I pretend that I trust them'. Which does this phenomenon represent?

A   A normal phenomenon
B   Autistic thinking
C   Circumstantiality
D   Thought alienation
E   Thought echo

102. 'The television newsreader was wearing a blue jacket to indicate that I was going to be taken ill'. Which does this phenomenon represent?

A   Delusion of infidelity
B   Delusion of love
C   Delusion of persecution
D   Delusion of poverty
E   Delusion of reference

103. 'I saw a black cat crossing the road and I immediately knew that the police were after me'. What does this phenomenon represent?

A   Delusion of control
B   Delusion of guilt
C   Delusion of persecution
D   Delusion of reference
E   Delusional perception

104. A 29-year-old man attended an outpatient clinic. The clinician asked him to raise his arms and stretch them out in front of him. He then pricked his palm. Every time the clinician asked, the patient obliged and the clinician pricked his palm. Which of the following describes this psychopathological sign?

A   Ambitendency
B   Automatic obedience
C   Catalepsy
D   Cooperation
E   Echopraxia

105. What is the most appropriate answer for the following statement?

'My brain is rotting and my heart has stopped beating.'

A   Delusion of control
B   Delusion of reference
C   Delusional perception
D   Hypochondriacal delusion
E   Nihilistic delusion

106. 'Parents are people who raise you. Anything that raises you can be a parent. Parents can be anything material, vegetable or mineral that has taught something'. What is the most likely speech disorder?

A   Echolalia
B   Echopraxia
C   Flight of ideas
D   Illogicality
E   Verbigeration

107. When a 59-year-old man with a chronic psychotic disorder was asked to describe an aeroplane and a boat he called them aero car and sea car respectively. What is the most likely speech disorder?

   A   Logoclonia
   B   Neologism
   C   Parapragmatism
   D   Para praxis
   E   *Vorbeireden*

108. A 21-year-old woman diagnosed with schizophrenia complained of hearing her thoughts aloud just before they occurred. What is this phenomenon called?

   A   Autoscopy
   B   *Écho de la pensée*
   C   Functional hallucination
   D   *Gedankenlautwerden*
   E   Hypnagogic hallucinations

109. A 27-year-old female graduate was admitted to a hospital in Edinburgh with a drug- induced psychosis. She reported that she heard her boyfriend in Swansea talking to her. What is the most likely phenomenon?

   A   Extracampine hallucination
   B   Functional hallucination
   C   Illusion
   D   Pseudo-hallucination
   E   Reflex hallucination

110. 'When I think, I tend to think hard and my neighbours and family can hear my thoughts.' What is this phenomenon called?

   A   Normal phenomenon
   B   Thought alienation
   C   Thought broadcast
   D   Thought echo
   E   Thought withdrawal

111. A 77-year-old woman had lived on her own since her husband died 5 years ago. Over the years she had hoarded a lot of unnecessary possessions. However, since her husband's death the situation had progressively got worse. Which of the following is the most appropriate description of her behaviour?

   A   Anankastic personality disorder
   B   Bibliomania
   C   Diogenes syndrome
   D   Impulse control disorder
   E   Syllogomania

DYNAMIC PSYCHOPATHOLOGY

112. Which of the following psychodynamic terms is used for the process of combining several concepts into a single image?

   A   Condensation
   B   Displacement

C   Dream work
D   Secondary elaboration
E   Symbolism

113. A 25-year-old woman repeatedly thought that her mother would fall ill and die in the near future. However, she regarded such thoughts as alien and intrusive ideas that had no real connection with her. They did not arouse guilt or feelings of wishfulness. Which of the following defence mechanisms can explain the situation?

A   Denial
B   Idealisation
C   Identification
D   Isolation
E   Sublimation

114. A 53-year-old man drank excessive alcohol for many years. He made a long and sustained recovery from alcohol dependence. He now regarded himself as a reformed alcoholic and obtained a great deal of satisfaction by helping others in the context of Alcoholics Anonymous. Which of the following coping mechanisms can explain this situation?

A   Altruism
B   Displacement
C   Intellectualisation
D   Rationalisation
E   Undoing

HISTORY OF PSYCHIATRY

115. How old was Phineas Cage when he sustained an injury to frontal part of his brain?

A   25 years
B   27 years
C   29 years
D   31 years
E   45 years

116. Who discovered lithium?

A   Cade
B   Cameron
C   Kahlbaum
D   Kane
E   Ribot

117. Who introduced electroconvulsive therapy?

A   Cerletti
B   Kane
C   Meduna
D   Ribot
E   Sakel

118. Which of the following was the first selective serotonin reuptake inhibitor to be developed and introduced into the market?

A   Citalopram
B   Fluoxetine
C   Paroxetine
D   Sertraline
E   Zimelidine

119. Who discovered the hypothesis that antipsychotics work largely by blocking dopamine receptors?

A   Carlsson and Linquist
B   Dale and Laidlaw
C   Delay and Deniker
D   Den Boer
E   John Kane

120. In which year was electroconvulsive therapy introduced in the UK?

A   1930
B   1934
C   1948
D   1950
E   1958

121. Who introduced the term 'law of effect', which basically considers reinforcement as the main driver of behaviour?

A   Bandura
B   Kohler
C   Pavlov
D   Skinner
E   Thorndike

122. Who is associated with the introduction of electroconvulsive therapy?

A   Biltz
B   Bini
C   Cade
D   Delay
E   Tuke

123. Which of the following concepts is associated with Margaret Mahler?

A   Anal phase
B   Concrete operational stage
C   Normal autism
D   Preconventional morality
E   Trust versus mistrust

BASIC ETHICS AND PHILOSOPHY OF PSYCHIATRY

124. Which of the following mental disorders in Japan was renamed Togo Schicco Sho (loss of coordination disorder) to combat the stigma associated with the illness?

A   Autism

     B   Bipolar affective disorder
     C   Borderline personality disorder
     D   Developmental coordination disorder
     E   Schizophrenia

125. What does the 'pathoplastic effect' refer to in the context of cultural psychiatry meaning?

     A   Culture causes the mental illness
     B   Culture contributes to the frequency of the psychopathology
     C   Culture contributes to the manifestation of the psychopathology
     D   Culture pathologises certain types of behaviours which are termed illness
     E   Culture causes the reactions to mental illness

126. Which of the following refers to the Genovese syndrome or the bystander effect?

     A   Bystanders are less likely to help the victim if more people are present
     B   Bystanders are more likely to help if the victim is a woman
     C   Bystanders encourage others to be more altruistic
     D   Bystanders have a general tendency to help victims
     E   The victim is ignored by people around him or her because they are worried about their own safety

STIGMA AND CULTURE

127. A 41-year-old Ethiopian man was 'possessed' by a spirit, hitting his head against the wall, shouting, singing, laughing and crying. From what is he most likely to suffer?

     A   Ghost sickness
     B   Hwabyung
     C   Mal de ojo
     D   Spell
     E   Zar

Answers: MCQs

1. E Recapitulation of information is encouraged

During a psychiatric interview, both verbal and non-verbal communications are important, and not only factual information elicited from the patient. Open questions are good to initiate an interview, allowing information to flow, and closed questions help to obtain factual information and specific details. The interviewer should have a balance on open questions (usually at the beginning) and closed questions (usually come up later in the interview). Questions should be simple. Polythematic questions usually confuse patients. It is helpful to summarise and recapitulate information during the interview when clarifying what has been shared.

2. E Vascular dementia

The terminology and concept of vascular dementia are currently becoming more controversial and uncertain. It is cited as the second commonest cause of dementia after Alzheimer's disease. However, there is a growing body of opinion challenging this entity as commonly understood. Although memory impairment is seen in vascular dementia the most characteristic deficits are those of frontal and subcortical dysfunction. It has been argued that the concept of vascular dementia should be replaced with one of vascular cognitive impairment, a much broader description encompassing all forms of cognitive dysfunction due to cerebrovascular disease. It is likely that pure Alzheimer's dementia and pure vascular dementia are rare entities, and the mixed pathology is far more common than previously thought.

3. A Circumstantiality

Clang association, circumstantiality, flight of ideas, neologism and tangentiality are all examples of formal thought disorders. Circumstantiality is the over-inclusion of irrelevant details before reaching the final answer. It is usually seen in patients with schizophrenia or mania.

4. D Russell's sign

This is primarily found in patients with bulimia nervosa. Xanthelasma is yellowish deposit of cholesterol under the skin, usually on or around the eyelid. It may be associated with hyperlipidaemia, ischaemic heart disease and diabetes mellitus. Osler's nodes, splinter haemorrhages and Janeway's lesions are due to infectious endocarditis in intravenous drug users. A Kayser–Fleischer ring is a golden-brown pigment around the cornea in Wilson's disease. Lanugo hair is found in people with anorexia nervosa.

Table 4.1 Characteristic signs in mental and physical disorders

Sign	Disorder	Characteristic
Kayser–Flescher ring	Wilson's disease	Golden-brown pigment around cornea
Lanugo	Anorexia nervosa malnourishment	Soft wool-like hair covering the body
Osler's nodes	Infective endocarditis in intravenous drug abusers	Other signs seen in infective endocarditis: Janeway's lesions, splinter haemorrhages
Russell's sign	Eating disorder: anorexia nervosa or bulimia nervosa	Calluses on the dorsum of the hand caused by self-induced vomiting or purging in a patient with an eating disorder
Xanthelasma	Hyperlipidaemia Ischaemic heart disease Diabetes mellitus	Yellowish deposit of cholesterol under the skin, usually on or around the eyelid

5. E Open question

The establishment of a therapeutic relationship is one of the most important aspects of the psychiatric interview, which involves establishing a rapport with the patient. In a psychiatric interview, it is advisable to start with open questions such as 'What brought you to the hospital today?' or 'How can I help you?'. This provides the patient with an opportunity to open up and speak more. The purpose of an open question is to gather as much information as possible in the initial stages of the interview.

6. B Compound question

Compound questioning style is considered to be one of the obstructive interventions when conducting a psychiatric interview. The interview is not just asking the questions but also includes a process of formulating to achieve differential diagnoses. Through the appropriate use of open and closed questions is possible to gather more information to refine the formulation and diagnosis.

7. B Clang association

It is a form of a formal thought disorder observed during the mental state examination. It is seen in thought rhyming or assonance. It is a repetition of identical or similar sounding vowels in adjustment words. Here the thoughts are associated with the sound of the word rather than its meaning.

8. A It does not assess frontal lobe functioning

The MMSE is a standard screening test for cognitive functions and was introduced by Folstein. It is a 30-point examiner-rated scale. A clinical interview is the best diagnostic tool for any disorder, including dementia, rather than the MMSE. It assesses temporal, occipital and parietal lobe function, but it does not examine frontal lobe functions. It is not a culturally sensitive and user-friendly test.

9. E Wisconsin card sorting test

This is a widely used test of set-shifting ability which is thought to be compromised in patients with frontal lobe damage. Raven's progressive matrices consist of a series of visuospatial problem-solving tasks. It is also a test that is used to assess parietal lobe functioning. The digit span is used to assess attention and concentration. The Rey–Osterrieth complex figure test is used to test visual memory.

10. D Rivermead behavioural memory test

Table 4.2 Memory tests	
Test	**Measurement and evaluation**
Auditory verbal learning test	Verbal learning and memory (ability to learn 'unrelated words' in a rote-learning fashion)
California verbal learning test	Verbal learning and memory (ability to learn 'related words' in a rote-learning fashion)
Digit span	Working memory capacity and attention (ability of patient to repeat words in forward and backward fashion)
Rivermead behavioural memory test	Detect impairment of everyday memory problems Monitoring of change during treatment (used in patients with acquired brain injury that is non-progressive in nature)
Wechsler memory scale – III	Auditory and visual memory – declarative and working (Most recent version is Wechsler memory scale – IV)

11. A Considerable amount of traumatic experience-related information is stored as situationally accessible memory

Two memory systems are important for the understanding of post-traumatic stress disorder (PTSD). Verbally accessible memory (VAM) is declarative and hippocampal dependent. Situationally accessible memory (SAM) is non-declarative and amygdala dependent. In PTSD, a considerable amount of traumatic information resides solely in the SAM system. SAM memories are vulnerable to reactivation by cues. VAM memory can be retrieved deliberately or automatically. It can be edited and incorporated into a person's autobiographical memory. Stress impairs VAM, whereas SAM is unaffected by it.

12. A Capgras' syndrome

In this syndrome, patients believe that an imposter has replaced a known person. Up to 40% of patients have an organic disorder such as head injury or dementia. Capgras' syndrome is a mirror image of prosopagnosia. Facial recognition involves two distinct routes such as one for facial identification and another for detection of emotional significance. In Capgras' syndrome, the person's face looks identical; however, the emotional feelings are affected. Patients with prosopagnosia have a defect in facial recognition.

13. B Wechsler test of adult reading

the Wechsler test of adult reading is an equivalent test to the national adult reading test (NART). It is a pronunciation test and has been co-normed with the Wechsler adult intelligence scale (WAIS). Tests such as WAIS, the Wechsler abbreviated scale of intelligence and the Wechsler intelligence scale for children are intelligence tests that measure current intelligence. The Cambridge cognitive examination is a neuropsychological test for assessing cognitive functions.

14. E Wisconsin card scoring test

This is a test of frontal executive functions. The doors and people test is a test of visual and verbal memory, which is assessed by recall and recognition. Rey's auditory verbal learning test is a useful test to assess semantic memory difficulties. The Rey–Osterrieth test is useful in assessing visuospatial constructional ability and visual memory. The Rivermead behavioural memory test is used in assessing memory functions, especially in brain-injured patients.

15. B Raven's progressive matrices

When a patient has language disorder or where English is not his first language, Raven's progressive matrices test can be used to assess the intelligence. It is based on inductive reasoning and there are no verbal instructions involved. In addition, it has an advanced version for people who function at a high range of ability. Non-English versions of WAIS-III and the Wechsler intelligence scale for children are not available. Stanford–Binet is another test for intelligence. The Bender gestalt test is a visuo-motor test used in children to assess the perceptual motor ability.

16. C 24 or less

The MMSE is a good screening tool for cognitive impairment. The maximum score in MMSE is 30. A score of 24 or less raises the possibility of dementia in older people, with at least 9 years of formal education. If a person has been high functioning then even with higher scores one should suspect cognitive dysfunction. A MMSE score of 30/30 does not rule out cognitive dysfunction.

17. B Diencephalic amnesia

Transient global amnesia is characterised by sudden onset of confusion, disorientation and loss of memory. The patient recovers within minutes or hours. It usually leaves a gap in the memory, i.e. focal memory loss. An acute closed head injury has a similar presentation but there is very limited retrograde amnesia and impaired attention. Patients with Korsakoff's syndrome or diencephalic amnesia have intact working memory. Short-term memory is affected by defects in memory coding. The retrograde memory loss may be extensive. Patients with hippocampal damage have problems with anterograde memory. Retrograde memory will be preserved. In terms of memory loss, transient epileptic amnesia features are similar to transient global amnesia.

18. E Wrist drop

This is a radial nerve palsy and is also called 'Saturday night palsy'. An individual falls asleep with the arm hanging over the back of the chair, which compresses the radial nerve in its course through the axilla. The radial nerve supplies the extensors of the wrist and paralysis of these muscles leads to the characteristic wrist drop. There is also a small area of anaesthesia in the web between the thumb and index finger over the dorsum of the hand.

19. A Calf pain

The lumbar disc is most likely to prolapse, in particular the lowest two. When a disc protrudes, it generally compresses the nerve roots numbered one inferior to the disc. Therefore, in L5–S1 prolapse, the S1 nerve is compressed. Calf pain, decreased ankle jerk, weak foot planter flexion and weak knee flexion are associated with such a presentation. Decreased sensation on the outer dorsum of the foot is consistent with L4–5 prolapse affecting nerve root L5.

20. B Bitemporal hemianopia

The patient presents with symptoms that could be consistent with a pituitary tumour. In the central visual pathway, the two optic nerves converge to form the optic chiasma, at which point the axons derived from the nasal portions of the two retinae decussate and pass into the contralateral optic tract. Compression of the optic chiasma by an adjacent pituitary tumour leads to bitemporal hemianopia.

21. B Contralateral homonymous hemianopia

The lateral medullary syndrome results from the occlusion of one vertebral artery or the posterior inferior cerebellar artery. The patient may have vomiting, dysphagia, vertigo, ipsilateral Horner's syndrome, crossed pattern sensory loss (analgesia to pin-prick on ipsilateral face and contralateral trunk and limbs), ipsilateral ataxia and nystagmus.

22. E Right middle cerebral artery occlusion

The middle cerebral artery supplies the lateral aspect of each hemisphere. Occlusion of this artery presents with:

- Contralateral hemiplegia and sensory loss mainly of the face and arm
- Dysphagia and dyspraxia (dominant hemisphere)
- Contralateral neglect (non-dominant hemisphere)
- Contralateral homonymous hemianopia.

23. C Dementia of Lewy bodies

The characteristic features of dementia of Lewy bodies are progressive cognitive decline, pronounced fluctuations in cognition and attention, recurrent visual hallucinations and parkinsonism. The vivid dreams represent a rapid eye movement sleep disorder.

24. E Somatisation disorder

In this scenario, the patient presents with a long history of several somatic complaints that have no identifiable physical cause. In addition, these symptoms have started before the age of 30 years. Hence, the most likely diagnosis is somatisation disorder. If the patient had presented with a fixed belief that the somatic complaints are indicative of serious illness and preoccupied with a diagnosis, the most likely diagnosis would have been hypochondriasis. In body dysmorphic disorder, the patient is preoccupied with one or more perceived defects that are either completely imagined or not significant. They spend a significant amount of time thinking about this defect/defects causing extreme distress and affecting their day-to-day life. Neurasthenia is characterised by chronic fatigue and weakness, both mental and physical, which is brought about by minimal physical or mental strain. Patients can present with generalised aches and pain. This diagnosis is described in the ICD-10 but is no longer in the DSM-IV. Malingering is intentionally feigning or exaggerating physical or psychological symptoms and/or illness for a clear external gain. The common theme in all the five options is that there is no medical cause identified on assessment and investigations.

25. D Opioids

The Ghodse opioid addiction test relies on the observation that naloxone eyedrops have no effect on the pupils of an opioid-naïve individual or an occasional opioid user. However, they cause dilatation of pupils if the individual is dependent on opioids.

26. D Practice effect

Halo effect is the tendency of a rater to overestimate a subject's response based on a prior assumption. Hawthorne effect is the non-specific effect caused by the knowledge subjects has that they are participating in an experimental study.

27. A Brief psychiatric rating scale

This is the oldest rating scale that is used to measure chronic psychotic symptoms. It is a semi-structured interview schedule with 18 items and some versions include up to 25 items. It rates conceptual disorganisation, hostility and social withdrawal. It is better for psychosis than for depression or anxiety.

28. B DAT scan

This scan involves the use of radio-isotopes to measure levels of dopamine in the brain. It works by binding to dopamine transporters in the brain, in particular the striatum. The DAT scan can assist in differentiating between Alzheimer's disease and dementia of the Lewy body. The characteristic histopathological feature of dementia of the Lewy body is the presence of Lewy bodies in the cerebral cortex. As in Parkinson's disease, they are also seen in the substantia nigra. Their composition is the same in both diseases. The key protein is α-synuclein, although routine detection of Lewy bodies is currently based on the presence of another protein, ubiquitin.

29. D Stage 2 of grief reaction

Bereavement is the loss through death of a loved one. Grief is the involuntary emotional and behavioural response to the bereavement. Mourning is the voluntary expression of behaviours and rituals that are socially sanctioned responses to bereavement. Grief is a continuous process, but for clarity it can be described as having three stages. Stage 1 lasts from a few hours to several days. Stage 2 usually lasts from a few weeks to about 6 months, but may be much longer. In stage 3, the symptoms subside and everyday activities are resumed.

30. D Migrated from other country

High rates of schizophrenia have been reported among some migrants. The reasons for these high rates in this population are not clear, but they may be due to disproportionate migration of people who are unsettled because they are becoming mentally ill. The effects of a new environment may also play a part in provoking illness in predisposed people.

31. C Cocaine use in pregnancy

The causes of violent behaviour among young people are not fully understood. Cocaine use in pregnancy has been associated with an increased risk of violence in children when there has been prenatal exposure to cocaine.

32. B 2–4 times higher

Panic disorder is a familial disorder. Rates in monozygotic twins are higher than in dizygotic twins, indicating that the family aggregation is due to genetic factors. The mode of inheritance is not known.

33. D Vitamin D

McGrath (1999) proposed a hypothesis that low vitamin D levels in mothers may increase the risk of adult-onset schizophrenia. It is postulated that deficiency of vitamin D in mothers may affect the fetal brain and overall neurodevelopment, increasing the risk of several illness, such as multiple sclerosis, schizophrenia. However, there is more research needed to establish a link between maternal deficiency of vitamin D and risk of adult-onset schizophrenia in the offspring.

34. A Decreases

Kendler et al (2001) have studied the association of genetic risk, number of previous depressive episodes and stressful life events with the onset of a major depressive episode following previous episodes:

1. High genetic risk of major depression – it was noted that patients with a high genetic risk of depression had spontaneous onset of the depressive episode with little to no association with stressful life events, irrespective of presence or absence of previous depressive episodes.
2. Low genetic risk of major depression – patients with a low genetic risk of major depression had onset of first depressive episode after a major stressful life event. However, as the number of depressive episodes increased, the association between life event and onset of another major depressive episode reduced. In summary, subsequent events of depressed episodes may occur spontaneously or after a lower level of stressful life events.

35. C Environmental cause

The exact cause of schizophrenia is not known. Genetics, birth complications, head injury, epilepsy and drug use increase the risk of schizophrenia by 2- to 4.5-fold. Andreasson et al, in a longitudinal study of Swedish conscripts, caused controversy by finding evidence to support the hypothesis that there are possible environmental causes of schizophrenia.

36. B January, February, March

The season of birth effect has been replicated in several studies that were carried out in the northern hemisphere. There appears to be a 5–15% excess in the winter and early spring. It has been reported that schizophrenia is more common in people born in the first 3 months of the year.

37. E Schizophrenia

Selten et al (2007) have suggested certain risk factors for schizophrenia, one of which is long-term exposure to the experience of social defeat. This may be due to the sensitisation of a mesolimbic neurotransmitter pathway, resulting in increased dopamine and thereby increased risk of schizophrenia. In addition, other risk factors for schizophrenia include lower intelligence, sensory deficits, living in an urban area, immigration form lower income countries and exposure to abuse. Low IQ or hearing deficits are also considered risk factors for schizophrenia.

38. E Schizotypal personality disorder

The characteristic features of schizotypal personality disorder include acute discomfort with close relationships, eccentricities of behaviour, and a range of cognitive or perceptual disorders.

Its incidence is slightly higher in men than in women. Its prevalence in the general population is estimated to be between 0.1% and 5.6%. It is frequently associated with personality disorders such as borderline, avoidant, paranoid and schizoid, which indicate that the diagnosis is underpinned by a taxon or discrete diagnostic entity.

39. E Schizophrenia

This is characterised by a fundamental disturbance of thinking, perception and affect that is inappropriate and blunted. In acute polymorphic psychotic disorder, delusions and hallucinations are markedly variable and change from day to day or even from hour to hour. Delirium tremens is an alcohol withdrawal state.

40. D Prodromal symptoms of psychotic disorder

Individuals developing a psychotic disorder experience prodromal symptoms such as social isolation, impairment of functioning, blunted affect, perceptual abnormalities such as illusions, sleep disturbances, speech abnormalities, and concentration and memory problems. The prodromal symptoms take an average of 6 months to manifest into a first psychotic episode.

41. E Social phobia

It is prevalent in males and peaks at age 5 and between 11 and 15 years. The individual with the condition usually does not present to services before 30 years of age. The presentation consists of somatic symptoms such as blushing and perspiration when exposed to a feared situation. Patients avoid situations thus leading to minimal social contact. They tend to look for jobs that are less demanding. Thoughts of suicide are common.

42. B Postschizophrenic depression

Disorganised schizophrenia, schizoaffective disorder and schizophreniform disorder are classified under schizophrenia and other psychotic disorders in the DSM-IV. Schizoaffective disorder is a separate category in the ICD-10. Schizotypal disorder is a separate category in the ICD-10 and is included under personality disorders in the DSM-IV.

43. E 1994

DSM	Publication year	ICD	Publication year
Table 4.3 The DSM and ICD classifications			
DSM-I	1952	ICD-6	1948
DSM-II	1968	ICD-8	1968
DSM-III	1980	ICD-9	1978
DSM-III R	1987	ICD-10	1992
DSM-IV	1994		
DSM-IV-TR	2000		
DSM-V	2013		

44. A Axis I

Until the publication of the DSM-IV in 1994, autistic disorder was categorised as an axis II disorder, which includes personality disorder and intellectual disabilities. However, in the DSM-IV, autistic disorder was categorised as an axis I disorder, which includes clinical disorders, such as major mental disorders, learning disorders and substance use disorders. The reason for this move is likely to be increased recognition that autistic disorders have a neurobiological and developmental origin. Also, symptoms of autistic disorder may vary and are at times responsive to intervention.

45. E Narcissistic personality disorder

Narcissistic personality disorder is completely absent from the ICD-10 classification system. This disorder is classified as a personality disorder in the DSM-IV. The equivalent disorders in the ICD-10 and DSM-IV are as follows:

Table 4.4 DSM-IV and ICD-10 personality disorders

ICD-10	DSM-IV
Anankastic	Obsessive–compulsive
Anxious	Avoidant
Dissocial	Antisocial
Histrionic	Histrionic

46. C 3 months

In cases of persistent delusional disorder, delusions are the most prevalent or possibly the only symptoms. The symptoms should have persisted for at least 3 months before a diagnosis can be made.

Table 4.5 Duration of symptoms required for an ICD-10 diagnosis

Diagnosis	Duration
Persistent delusional disorder	Symptoms for at least 3 months and should be clearly personal rather than subcultural
Depression	Depressive symptoms/episode for at least 2 weeks
Schizophrenia	Symptoms for at least 1 month or more
Post-traumatic stress disorder	Onset of symptoms after the trauma within few weeks to months, but before 6 months. Rarely after 6 months
Schizotypal disorder	Typical features should have been present, continuously or episodically, for at least 2 years

47. C Other neurotic disorder

Neurasthenia is included in the ICD-10 but not the DSM-IV. It is commonly diagnosed in far eastern countries. Conversion disorder is a somatoform disorder.

48. C Mixed and other personality disorder

The category of other disorders of adult personality and behaviour includes diagnostic categories that do not fit neatly into other categories.

49. D Transient stress-related paranoid ideation

Borderline personality disorder was originally used to describe individuals with instability. In the DSM-IV, there is an additional criterion, not mentioned in the ICD-10, of transient paranoia.

50. E 24 months

The diagnostic criteria for cyclothymia involve several periods of depression and mania with or without intervening periods of normal moods. The episodes of depression and mania are not severe enough to meet the criteria of a manic or depressive episode.

51. C Olanzapine

The most robust data support the effectiveness of amisulpride in primary negative symptoms but even this effect seems no better than haloperidol. A well-conducted study appeared to show superiority for olanzapine over amisulpride.

52. D 60–70% with selective serotonin reuptake inhibitors

Prevalence of side effects in antidepressants is listed below:

Tricyclic antidepressants 30%
Selective serotonin reuptake inhibitors 60–70%
Monoamine oxidase inhibitors 40%
Venlafaxine 70%
Trazodone unknown
Mirtazapine 25%
Reboxetine 5–10%
Duloxetine 46%

53. E Ziprasidone

The most common side effect, namely sedation, was observed in four of five antipsychotics in clinical antipsychotic trials of the intervention effectiveness study. These four drugs were olanzapine, risperidone, quetiapine and perphenazine. Ziprasidone was not associated with an increased side effect of sedation.

54. E Naltrexone

The National Institute for Health and Care Excellence (NICE) recommends the use of naltrexone for those who prefer an abstinence programme. Patients need to be fully informed of the potential adverse effects and benefits of treatment, and should be highly motivated to remain on treatment. Naltrexone treatment has been found by NICE to be a cost-effective treatment strategy in aiding abstinence from opioid misuse.

55. B Naltrexone acts on all three types of opioid receptors

It is an opioid antagonist acting on all three types of receptors, namely, μ, δ and κ receptors. In opiate-dependent individuals administration of naltrexone causes a rise in blood pressure. It is a relatively long-acting drug. Use of naltrexone is not associated with a reduced risk of suicide in opiate-dependent individuals.

56. E N-Methyl-D-aspartate receptor antagonism

Acamprosate is used in alcohol-dependent patients to maintain abstinence. It is supposed to reduce craving. The possible mechanisms of action are N-methyl-D-aspartate receptor antagonism and γ-aminobutyric acid A receptor agonism. Effects on D_2 and $5-HT_2$ receptors are not clear.

57. C α_2-Receptor antagonism

Clozapine has marked anticholinergic activity. It acts as a muscarinic receptor blocker except for M_4-receptor agonism. This is likely to cause hypersalivation. In addition α_2-receptor antagonism could increase salivation. Dopamine receptor blockade and $5-HT_2$ antagonism explain the antipsychotic property and α_1-receptor blockade leads to hypotension.

58. C $5-HT_3$

This receptors are G-protein-coupled metabotrophic receptors with the exception of the $5-HT_3$-receptor, which is a ligand-gated ion channel receptor. It has five subunits and affects the transmission of sodium, potassium and calcium. When serotonin binds to a $5-HT_3$-receptor, it leads to an increase in intracellular calcium. This activation of the receptor leads to receptor excitation and neurotransmission. These receptors are present on both pre- and postsynaptic nerve terminals.

Presynaptic $5-HT_3$-receptors are known to mediate and modulate various neurotransmitters

Postsynaptic $5-HT_3$-receptors are present in the caudate nucleus, putamen, hippocampus and amygdala. When activated, postsynaptic receptors lead to fast and excitatory neurotransmission.

59. A Clozapine

This competitively inhibits $5-HT_3$-receptors. Other antipsychotics mentioned in the question inhibit this receptor in a non-competitive fashion.

60. A Antabuse irreversibly blocks aldehyde dehydrogenase

On discontinuation of Antabuse for alcohol dependence, it can take up to 2 weeks for a person to synthesise new enzymes that metabolise alcohol. Therefore, patients who are on Antabuse are advised not to drink for up to 2 weeks after stopping alcohol.

61. E Wilson's disease

This patient has clinical features suggestive of Wilson's disease. It is associated with a defective metabolism and accumulation of copper in the body. The affected individual develops cirrhosis and Kayser–Fleischer rings in the cornea. They can present with involuntary movements.

62. B Chemical antagonism

Chelation is an example of chemical antagonism. Copper is chelated by D-penicillamine and urinary excretion of copper is increased.

63. C 15 hours

Lithium is rapidly and completely absorbed with serum concentrations peaking in 1–1½ hours. The elimination half-life of lithium is between 18 and 24 hours. Lithium is mainly excreted by the kidneys. Some excretion also takes place through faeces and sweat.

64. C Lithium

Most drugs undergo metabolism before excretion. Lithium is excreted unchanged in the urine.

65. E Tremor

Fine tremor is an acute side effect of lithium therapy. Coarse tremor is a sign of lithium toxicity. Other options in the question are chronic side effects of long-term therapy with lithium.

66. E Reciprocal inhibition

This is a phenomenon used in relaxation therapy for anxiety disorder and in systemic desensitisation. In this, if a stimulus with an undesired response such as anxiety, and a stimulus with a desired response such as relaxations, are presented together, their incompatibility will result in a reduction to the undesired response.

67. A Aversive conditioning

Aversion therapy is used mainly in conditions with drug and alcohol addiction. Here the unconditional stimulus is an unpleasant stimulus and it is paired with the target behaviour.

Antabuse (unconditional stimulus) + alcohol = nausea (conditional response)

Alcohol = nausea (conditional response) = avoidance of alcohol.

68. B Classic conditioning

Before conditioning:

i. Waiting in the waiting area   → No panic attacks
ii. Fear of exposure to the needle   → Panic attack

During conditioning:

iii. Waiting in the waiting area + fear → Panic attack

After conditioning:

iv. Waiting in waiting area   → Panic attack.

69. B Extinction

Repeated exposure to the conditioned stimulus without the unconditioned stimulus results in a gradual weakening of the conditional response, and eventually results in stopping the conditional response. This is called extinction. In other words, it is the unlearning of behaviour and occurs when behaviour is not reinforced over a period of time.

Flooding and implosion are the techniques used in the treatment of phobic disorders.

70. C Catastrophic thinking

This is an irrational thought that leads to the belief that something is far worse than it actually is. Concentrating on the worst-case scenario or outcome of a situation is known as catastrophic thinking. Black- and-white thinking is also called dichotomous thinking, where a person thinks all or none and does not accept any other possibilities. Selective abstraction is described as focusing on one aspect of an event and ignoring the more important features. Maximisation and minimisation are exaggerating or overtly reducing the importance of the events respectively.

71. D Overgeneralisation

Application of conclusions on the wider range of events or situations, which are based on one or isolated experience is known as overgeneralisation. In this scenario, the young doctor could be good in other aspects of life such as interpersonal relationships. Arbitrary inference is described as drawing a conclusion in the absence of sufficient evidence. Personalisation is described as relating an external event to oneself.

72. E Personalisation

This refers to relating external events to oneself when there is no particular reason to do so. All events that can be brought into consciousness are associated with a sense of personal possession, although this is not usually in the forefront of consciousness. This 'I' quality has been called personalisation: and may be disturbed in psychological disorders. There are two aspects to the sense of self-activity/personalisation; the sense of existence and the awareness of the performance of one's actions. The individual blames him- or herself for the consequences of others' actions. In this scenario, the treating doctor is personalising the death of an elderly patient who had a sudden cardiac arrest and a poor prognosis.

73. A Arbitrary inference

This refers to drawing a conclusion in the absence of sufficient evidence. Cognitive distortions or biases are characterised by systemic logical errors in thinking. In this particular case, the young girl believes that her boyfriend is cheating on her, even in the absence of such evidence.

74. C 4 months

Vision is the least developed of the senses in an infant. Infants can track and scan objects, and see faces at a distance of 25–50 cm. At 1 month, infants can scan external features of a face and a preference is shown for complex stimuli. At 2 months, infants possess the ability to visualise the three-dimensional representation of a face, and can focus on the internal features of the face such as the eyes and mouth. By 3 months of age, infants are able to recognise photographs of their mother's face. At 4 months, colour vision and accommodation have developed. At 6 months, visual acuity almost reaches the adult level and is complete by 3 years.

75. C Initiative versus guilt

According to Erikson, psychological development continues throughout life through the eight stages. Each person is thought to go through the stages in the same order and each stage has favourable and unfavourable outcomes.

1. Trust versus mistrust (birth to 18 months)
2. Autonomy versus shame (18 months to 3 years)
3. Initiative versus guilt (3–5 years)
4. Industry versus inferiority (6–11 years)
5. Identity versus role confusion (12–18 years)
6. Intimacy versus isolation (20–40 years)
7. Generativity versus stagnation (40–60 years)
8. Integrity versus despair (65+ years)

76. A Conventional: 13–16 years

Kohlberg's stages of moral development are described as follows:

1. **Preconventional:** 7–12 years to middle childhood; stage1: obedience and punishment orientation; stage 2: reward orientation
2. **Conventional:** 13–16 years; stage 3: good boy/good girl orientation; stage 4: maintaining social order and law
3. **Postconventional:** 16–20 years; stage 5: social contracts and individual rights; stage 6: universal principles of justice

77. B Attachment is increased if the mother is hostile towards her child

Children normally form an attachment to a primary caregiver from about 1–3 months of age who is not necessarily the mother (though usually). Multiple attachments can be formed even before 18 months. John Bowlby developed the concept of attachment theory. Attachment is increased, although it is insecure in type if the mother is hostile towards her children and anxious. In Harlow's monkey experiment, the infants ran to the terry cloth mother when their attachment system was activated by loud noises.

78. D Lorenz described newly hatched goslings programmed to follow a movable object

Imprinting is associated with Konrad Lorenz. He experimented showing that goslings responded to him as their mother. The concept is used to understand early developmental experiences on later life behaviours. Imprinting implies that, during a certain short period of development, a young animal is highly sensitive to a certain stimulus which then, but not at other times, provokes a specific behaviour pattern. Martin Seligman is associated with learned helplessness.

79. D It is an encouragement to explore and engage in a lot of play acts

This is an actual physical alignment in peer-reared monkeys to stressful situations in socially deprived non-human primates. The primates grasp each other in a clingy manner. The peers find it difficult to engage in exploratory play. The phenomenon has nothing to do with locomotive engines. Longitudinal studies in animal research have relevance to human behaviour and psychopathology.

80. D It increases when the onset of the mental disorder is acute

Aggressive behaviour assumes both violent and non-violent forms against others. Such behaviour increases when the onset of the mental disorder is acute. Aggression implies that there is an intent to harm or otherwise injure a person.

81. D It is a conditioned stimulus is constantly repeated without the unconditioned stimulus

JB Watson is associated with the concept of extinction. It predates partial recovery. A conditioned response may not be completely destroyed, because there may be a partial recovery if the animal is rested. Extinction occurs when the conditioned stimulus is constantly repeated without the unconditioned stimulus, until the response diminishes before disappearing.

82. B BF Skinner

BF Skinner: operant conditioning
JB Watson: extinction
Ivan Pavlov: classic conditioning
Albert Bandura: social learning
EL Thorndicke: law of effect

83. A Antilocution

Allport described five stages of prejudice and discrimination as follows:

1. Antilocution (name calling, stereotyping, can be done through humour)
2. Avoidance (exclusion)
3. Discrimination (refusal of service or denial of opportunity)
4. Physical attack (threat of physical violence, murder)
5. Extermination (genocide).

The above stages are progressive and have been repeatedly acted out throughout history in a set way. The progression of each stage will start with simple name calling, which then develops into stereotyping a group, which can then lead to defamation by exclusion and eventually avoidance. 'We don't have people like that in our club.'

84. C Instrumental function

In 1938, Daniel Katz proposed a functionalist theory of attitudes. Attitudes are determined by the functions for which they serve and are fairly resistant to change. Katz distinguished four types of psychological functions that attitudes meet, such as:

1. **Instrumental:** we develop favourable attitudes towards things that aid or reward us. People will favour a political party that will advance their own economic interests. It could also provide us with social approval from those whom we regard as important.
2. **Knowledge:** people seek a degree of order, clarity and stability in their personal frame of reference. Attitudes such as stereotypes bring order and clarity to the complexities of human life.
3. **Value-expressive:** these express our basic values, reinforcing our self-image. We may have a self-image of ourselves as a quirky Aquarius or a friendly northerner, and we cultivate attitudes that we believe indicate such a core value.

4. **Ego-defensive:** some attitudes serve to protect us from acknowledging the basic truth about ourselves and the harsh realities of life. They serve to protect our self-concept.

Accuracy function is not part of the functional theory.

85. A California Personality Inventory

Personality can be defined as the totality of a person's emotional and behavioural traits which characterise his or her day-to-day living. Personality disorders are deeply ingrained, maladaptive patterns of behaviour, generally recognisable by adolescence and continuing throughout adult life. The California Personality Inventory is valuable in enabling a complex picture of an individual to be derived, based on the profiles of scores on different scales. The general health questionnaire is used to determine psychiatric 'caseness' in epidemiological studies. The present state examination is a semi-structured interview with probes for each symptom and a detailed list of signs to be evaluated. It covers only the past 4 weeks, unless augmented by additional duration questions. The Montgomery–Asberg depression rating scale (MADRS) (10 items) is a depression rating scale designed to be sensitive to treatment changes. A limitation of the MADRS is the lack of a structured interview, which may affect its reliability.

86. D It is low for antisocial personality disorder

Reliability is a means to an end rather than an end in itself. Its importance lies in the fact that it sets a ceiling for validity. The lower it is the worse the validity becomes. Using a standardised interview can achieve considerably higher diagnostic reliability than is possible with unstructured interviews. It can be further improved by adopting operational definitions for all diagnostic categories. Organic and psychotic disorders generally have higher reliability than neurosis and personality disorders. This is probably due to the frequency of neurotic symptoms and maladaptive personality traits in the general population.

87. E Understanding of the origin and adoption of unhelpful 'modes'

Schema – focused models – are useful in the treatment of personality disorders. Understanding of the origin and adoption of unhelpful 'modes' of behaviour is a central feature of this model.

88. D Radical acceptance

Linehan et al (1994) developed this treatment for patients with borderline personality disorder who repeatedly harm themselves. Despite the name, it uses cognitive and behavioural techniques. It lasts up to 1 year. Individual therapy sessions contain four elements.

- Cognitive–behavioural techniques
- Dialectical ways of thinking about problems such as seeing causality in terms of both, rather than either/or, and also the possibility of reconciling opposites
- 'Mindfulness' which is the practice of detachment from experience
- Aphorism which is phrases that encapsulate the approach, e.g. although people may not have caused all their problems, they have to solve them anyway.

89. D Rolling with resistance

The key principles of motivational interviewing includes expressing empathy, developing discrepancy, rolling with resistance and supporting self-efficiency. The key stages in the transtheoretical model are precontemplation, contemplation, preparation, action, maintenance and termination.

90. E Systemic family therapy

In this therapy, hypothesising is used by the therapist to frame preliminary explanations of symptoms to the family. Circular questioning refers to the use of feedback to the therapist's questions to frame the next question; it is used to facilitate alternative explanations to the presenting problem.

91. C Cognitive–analytic therapy

The sequential diagrammatic reformulation is a schematic diagram with individuals' reciprocal role procedures deployed by individuals in specific situations.

92. E Random screening of drivers for breath alcohol levels is a form of primary prevention

Primary prevention is an attempt to reduce the incidents of new cases of problems in a general population. The random screening of drivers' breath alcohol by police is intended to prevent drinking and driving. Educating pregnant woman and teenagers about the hazards of substance misuse is an example of primary prevention. The continuation of mood stabilisers/antimanic drugs in patients with bipolar affective disorder is intended to prevent relapse and recurrences in these patients. This is an example of secondary prevention.

93. E Topiramate

Antipsychotics are used in as many as 50% of bipolar patients for long-term management. Some patients taking lithium have regular manic upswings that can be managed by giving oral antipsychotics for a few weeks. Anticonvulsants such as carbamazepine, valproate and lamotrogine are useful in the management of bipolar affective disorder and can prevent episodes of major depression.

94. B Fostering moderate informal drinking and promoting awareness of hazards

Primary prevention is aimed at reducing the prevalence of hazardous drinking or in some cases the hazards of drinking. It can be achieved by controls of availability, education, which needs to take into account the medium, the audience and the message, and provision of alternatives (promotion of low-alcohol beers and wines has proved helpful).

95. D Lithium

Most psychotropic drugs can produce fetal malformations when administered to pregnant laboratory animals. The possible translation of such data to humans led at one time to considerable concern. No specific increase in risk can be attributed to high-potency antipsychotics or tricyclics. Low-potency antipsychotics impart a small but significant increase in the risk of organ dysgenesis. Lithium is associated with a rate of Epstein's anomaly that is 400 times that of the general population. Valproate imparts a 2% risk of hypospadias. Carbamazepine is associated with a risk of spina bifida in the region of 0.5–1%. Benzodiazepines may be associated with a two fold increase in the risk of oral cleft abnormalities.

96. B It is associated with an unpleasant emotional state

Depersonalisation is defined as a subjective state of unreality in which there is a feeling of estrangement, either from a sense of self or from the external environment. The individual feels as if 'he is unreal'. The affected individual expresses uncertainty and paints a picture; 'as off' is the best way to describe it. Depersonalisation is subjective and unpleasant. It is invariably associated with emotional numbing and changes in the body: visual, auditory, tactile, gustatory or olfactory modalities. Loss of feeling of agency, disturbed body image and altered perception of time are reported.

97. B It has been demonstrated in animal experiments

In learned helplessness tasks, the organism initially receives non-contingent punishment in which the aversive stimulus is received irrespective of the animal's response. The contingency is then changed such that a response would lead to escape from the aversive stimulus, but the typical finding is that the animal remains helpless and does not find the escape response. Seligman proposed that learned helplessness could provide a model for the acquisition and maintenance of depression in human beings. He also proposed that depressed patients usually have attributional styles that are internal, stable and global. 'Internal' means that patients make causal attributions to internal personal traits rather than external events.

98. C Occur in Ganser's syndrome

Pseudo-hallucinations are defined in different ways. They are also used to describe hallucination-like experiences that take place in subjective space. Jasper identified a pseudo-hallucination as similar to a normal perception, except that it occurs in inner subjective space. Such hallucinations are not pathognomonic of any particular mental illness. They can be identified in the visual, auditory or tactile modality.

99. E Severe interference with social functioning

The symptom of hypomania is less intense than mania. Although patients with hypomania can present with elevated mood, pressure of speech, increased energy and irritability, it is not as severe as in mania. At times, it may be difficult to differentiate mania and hypomania. A mild degree of social and occupational interference may be present in hypomania. If delusions, hallucinations, and severe degree of interference with social and/or occupational functioning are present, it is indicative of mania.

100. D Running commentary

Hallucinatory voices vary in quality, ranging from those that are quite clear and can be ascribed to specific individuals to those that are vague and that the patient cannot describe with any clarity. In some cases, the voices speak about the person in the third person and may give a running commentary on their actions. These are among Schneider's first symptoms of schizophrenia.

101. A A normal phenomenon

'Autistic' thinking or undirected fantasy is quite common but certain people, when faced with repeated disappointing or adverse life circumstances, may engage in excessive undirected fantasy thinking. Circumstantiality occurs when thinking proceeds slowly with many unnecessary and trivial details, but finally the point is reached. The goal of thinking is never completely lost and thinking proceeds towards it by an intricate and convoluted path. In thought alienation, patients believe that their thoughts are under the control of an outside agency or that others are participating in their thinking. In thought echo, i.e. *écho de la pensée*, the patient hears them after the thoughts have occurred. When the patient hears his or her thoughts spoken just before or at the same time as they occur it is called *gedankenlautwerden*.

102. E Delusion of reference

This describes a situation in which the patient feels paranoid, the world becomes devoid of coincidence, and every incidental occurrence is referred directly to the patient and has a personal significance for them, usually implying threat. The patient finds hints and double meanings in perfectly ordinary statements or events. The patient believes that things are done in a special way to convey a meaning and situations are specially arranged to test them out.

103. E Delusional perception

This is the attribution of a new meaning, usually in the sense of self-reference to a normally perceived object or event. The new meaning cannot be understood as arising from the patient's affective state or previous attitudes. It must not be confused with delusional misinterpretation in which the delusional system affects all aspects of the patient's life, and so every event or perception is interpreted as being involved with that delusion.

104. B Automatic obedience

Some abnormally induced movements can be regarded as the result of undue compliance on the part of the patient, whereas others may be interpreted as indicating rejection of the environment. In automatic obedience, the patient carries out every instruction regardless of the consequence. 'Command automatism' is a synonym for automatic obedience. It occurs most commonly in catatonia, although it is also occasionally seen in dementia.

105. E Nihilistic delusion

This is also known as delusion of negation and it refers to the condition when patients deny the existence of their body, mind, loved ones and the world around them. This delusion occurs in the context of severe agitated depression, schizophrenia and delirium. Sometimes, it is associated with delusion of enormity when the patient believes that he or she can produce a catastrophe by some action.

106. D Illogicality

This is a form of thought disorder, in which there is intrinsic disagreement in thinking; it can lead to faulty conclusions. Illogicality may indicate schizophrenia. It can be present even though there is no delusional thinking.

107. B Neologism

The term 'neologism' is usually applied to new formations produced by patients with schizophrenia. It means new because the patient constructs words or ordinary words to be used in a new way. Neologisms in individuals with catatonia may be mannerisms or stereotypes. The patient may distort the pronunciations of some words in the same way as he or she distorts some body movements. Some patients use a stock word instead of the correct one. Malapropisms are conspicuously misused words, which may be mistaken for neologisms in some individuals, but they are of no particular known psychiatric significance.

108. D *Gedankenlautwerden*

Hearing one's own thoughts spoken aloud is a Schneider's first-rank symptom. Gedankenlautwerden describes hearing one's thoughts spoken just before or at the same time as they are occurring. *Écho de la pensée* is the phenomenon of hearing one's own thoughts after they have occurred.

109. A Extracampine hallucination

This is a hallucination that is outside the limits of the sensory field. These hallucinations can occur in healthy people as hypnagogic hallucinations but also in schizophrenia and organic disorders. A functional hallucination requires the presence of another real sensation. Patients can distinguish both features and crucially the hallucination does not occur without the stimulus. Functional hallucinations are not uncommon in chronic schizophrenia. Illusions are misperceptions of external stimuli, which are the transformation of perceptions, coming about by a mixing of the reproduced perceptions of the person's fantasy with natural perceptions. There are three types of illusion: completion illusion, affect illusion and pareidolia. Reflex hallucination, i.e. synaesthesia, is the experience of a stimulus in one sense modality producing a sensory experience in another.

110. A Normal phenomenon

A hallucination is a perception without an object, i.e. it represents perceptual deception. Hallucinations can be the result of intense emotions or a mental disorder, suggestion, sensory deprivation, and disorders of sense organs and the central nervous system. Thought alienation, thought broadcasting, thought echo and thought withdrawal are Schneider's first-rank symptoms, which are diagnostic of schizophrenia.

111. E Syllogomania

Some elderly people seem to become, by choice, reclusive and eccentric in old age and could end up living in squalor. Various names have been used to describe these patients, such as senile squalor syndrome and diogenes syndrome. A related, probably obsessive, problem of compulsive collecting, which can also lead to squalor, is called syllogomania. It is likely that elderly people may live in squalor for a variety of reasons, such as unrecognised physical illness, frontal lobe dysfunction, early dementia or other brain disease, depression, alcohol or drug abuse and life-long eccentric personality.

112. A Condensation

Dream work is a mental process for converting a latent dream (unconscious content of dream) into manifest contents (dream as experienced by the person).

Displacement is where desires and emotions are displaced from the intended person/object onto a meaningless object.

In condensation, several objects/concepts are combined into a single image.

Symbolism is the transformation of thought into sensory or symbolic image.

Secondary elaboration: refers to linking the separate elements of the dream into a coherent and more realistic story.

113. D Isolation

This is also known as intellectualisation and refers to a defence mechanism for coping with painful affects. The affect is separated from its contents, often treating it objectively rather than experientially. In a clinical setting, isolation is most commonly noted when the patient talks about his or her problems in an intelligent overly abstract manner and has difficulty describing, recalling and experiencing these feelings.

114. A Altruism

Coping mechanisms are considered to be on a somewhat higher adaptational level than defence mechanisms. Although coping mechanism may also ward off unpleasant or unconscious emotions and experiences, they are usually productive and helpful to both the patient and those around him or her. Altruism involves taking negative experience and turning it into a socially useful or positive one.

115. A 25 years

Phineas Gage was 25 years of age when he was involved in an accident. While he was working, there was an explosion that resulted in an iron rod being lodged in his head. He survived the accident. However, there was damage to his frontal lobes. After the accident, his personality and behaviour changed considerably.

116. A Cade

John FJ Cade was the first psychiatrist to discover lithium for the treatment of mania. He was Australian. The US Food and Drug Agency (FDA) approved this drug in 1970 for the treatment of mania. It is used for the short-term, long-term and prophylactic treatment of bipolar affective disorder.

117. A Cerletti

Cerletti and Bini conducted the first electrical induction of seizures in a patient with catatonia in 1938. Before this, the seizures were introduced chemically. Meduna (1934) used camphor to produce seizures in 1934. In 1940, electroconvulsive therapy was introduced in the USA. Sakel introduced 'insulin coma treatment' for schizophrenia in 1933.

118. E Zimelidine

The first selective serotonin reuptake inhibitor (SSRI) was zimelidine. Launched in 1981. But it was quickly withdrawn from the market due to an association with flu-like symptoms and Guillain–Barré syndrome. Fluoxetine was the second SSRI introduced successfully on the market in 1987.

119. A Carlsson and Linquist

In 1988, Den Boer found out that the SSRI fluvoxamine is effective in panic disorder. Kane et al (1987) stated that clozapine might be effective in resistant schizophrenia. Dale and Laidlaw (1910) described the action of histamine. Carlsson and Linquist developed the hypothesis that antipsychotics worked largely by blocking dopamine receptors in 1963. Delay and Deniker (1952) reported the effects of promethazine in psychosis.

120. B 1934

Convulsive therapy was introduced in 1934 by the Hungarian neuropsychiatrist Ladislas J Meduna (1934). Electroconvulsive therapy was invented in Italy and was used for the first time in the UK in 1939. Before 1939, seizures were artificially induced by cardiazol, also known as metrazol, in the mental hospitals in Britain.

121. E Thorndike

Bandura (1977) introduced the concept of observational learning, i.e. a novel behaviour develops by observational learning. Pavlov (1927) paired the conditioned and unconditioned stimuli and demonstrated various types of classic conditioning. Kohler, who was a major supporter of gestalt theory, believed that a problem would be solved once the 'missing piece of information' were found by perceptual restructuring of the elements constituting the problem (insight learning). He did not agree that past experiences affect the learning process. Skinner (1938) was the first behaviourist to describe operant conditioning. Thorndike (1998) came up with the 'law of effect', i.e. what happens as a consequence of any behaviour will determine the future of that behaviour.

122. B Bini

Ugo Cerletti and Lucio Bini administered the first electroconvulsive treatment in Rome in 1938. The major problems were patients' discomfort caused by the procedure and the bone fractures resulting from the motor activity of the seizure. Abraham Bennett (an American psychiatrist) helped develop the method of extracting pure curare from plant material, which led to the development of muscle relaxants to prevent fractures during ECT.

123. C Normal autism

The autistic phase is part of Mahler's separation–individuation theory. Margaret Mahler proposed this theory to describe how young children acquire a sense of identity separate from that of their mothers. The first 2 months are described as the normal autism stages, which consist of periods of sleep that outweigh periods of arousal in a state reminiscent of intrauterine life. The other stages include: symbiosis (2–5 months), differentiation (5–10 months), practising (10–18 months), rapprochement (18–24 months) and object constancy (2–5 years).

124. E Schizophrenia

The earlier names, 'seishi buntetsu byo' (split-mind disorder) to 'togo shiccho sho' (loss of coordination disorder), were said to be highly stigmatising and only 20% of the patients were told of their diagnosis by their doctors. The previous term went against the grain of traditional, culturally valued concepts of personal autonomy.

125. C Culture contributes to the manifestation of psychopathology

Terms in cultural psychiatry with their meanings are listed in **Table 4.6**.

Table 4.6 Position of culture-related syndromes	
Term	**Explanation**
Pathofacilitating	Culture contributes to the frequency of psychopathology
Pathogenic effect	Culture causes the mental illness
Pathoplastic effect	Culture contributes to the manifestation of psychopathology
Pathoreactive	Culture reactions to mental illness

126. A Bystanders are less likely to help the victim if more people are present

The bystander effect or genovese syndrome refers to the phenomenon the probability of individuals providing help to a victim in the presence of bystanders. According to this effect/syndrome, individuals do not intervene and do not help a victim if there are bystanders at the site of the emergency incident. It highlights that the more the number of bystanders, the less likely is an individual to provide help to the victim. This may be due to curiosity to look at others' reactions, perceiving the situation to be less urgent or allowing someone else to intervene and help the victim.

127. E Zar

This is a condition in which a person experiences being possessed by spirits. It may present as a dissociative episode and include singing, shouting, laughing, crying or head butting a wall. Patients may show apathy, withdrawal, or refusal to eat or do daily tasks. They may develop a relationship with the possessing spirit. Ghost sickness is seen in Native American tribes where the sufferer presents with weakness, bad dreams, fainting, anxiety, hallucination, confusion and feelings of suffocation. *Hwabyung* (also known as *wool-hwabyung*) is a Korean culture-bound syndrome, means 'anger syndrome' and is due to suppression of anger. There are symptoms of insomnia, fatigue, panic, dyspnoea and a feeling of an epigastric mass. *Mal de ojo* is a Spanish phrase which in English means 'evil eye', and is a concept in Mediterranean cultures in which the children have fitful sleep, cry for no reason, and have diarrhoea and vomiting with fever. It sometimes happens in adults, mainly women. *Spell* is a trance state when a person communicates with deceased relatives or spirits. It occurs among African–Americans and European Americans from South America.

Chapter 5

Mock examination

Questions: MCQs

For each question, select one answer option.

1. When assessing an angry and agitated patient, which of the following measures is advised?

    A   Avoid panic alarms because this irritates the patient
    B   Consider taking notes after the assessment has been completed
    C   Let the patient sit between interviewer and the door
    D   See the patient alone to allow disclosures of sensitive information
    E   Stay as close as possible to the patient so that he or she feels secure

2. When are closed questions most useful during a clinical assessment?

    A   At the start of an interview
    B   During the middle of unstructured interviews
    C   To control an overtalkative patient during the assessment
    D   When a chaperone presents during the assessment
    E   When the patient accepts the situation and starts crying during the assessment

3. If the psychiatrist asked a patient, 'Have you been feeling low in your mood recently?', what type of questioning style was used during the psychiatric interview?

    A   Closed question
    B   Compound question
    C   Directive question
    D   Leading question
    E   Open question

4. If the psychiatrist said to a patient 'You were not happy at that time?' what type of questioning style was used during the psychiatric interview?

    A   Closed question
    B   Compound question
    C   Directive question
    D   Leading question
    E   Open question

5. If the psychiatrist asked a patient 'tell me more about it?' What type of questioning style did he use during the psychiatric interview?

    A   Closed question
    B   Compound question
    C   Directive question
    D   Leading question
    E   Open question

6. Which lobe function is tested when the patient is asked to copy interlocking pentagons?

   A   Dorsolateral prefrontal cortex
   B   Frontal lobe
   C   Occipital lobe
   D   Parietal lobe
   E   Temporal lobe

7. In the mini-mental state examination (MMSE), what does the task of naming three objects test?

   A   Attention
   B   Concentration
   C   Orientation
   D   Recall
   E   Registration

8. A 45-year-old man had been drinking almost 35 units of alcohol a week for the last 7 years. He had numerous physical health and social difficulties. He understood that alcohol had become a problem in his life and was motivated to take help from alcohol services to stop it. What is the level of insight that he currently has?

   A   Action
   B   Intellectual insight
   C   Contemplation
   D   Ready for action
   E   True insight

9. Which of the following tests uses ambiguous stimuli to evaluate a person's patterns of thought, attitudes and observational capacity, and emotional responses?

   A   Cattell's personality factor questionnaire
   B   Minnesota multiphasic personality inventory 2
   C   Rey–Osterrieth complex figure test
   D   Rorschach's inkblot test
   E   Stanford–Binet test

10. A 72-year-old man was unable to draw interlocking polygons. Which of the following cerebral lobes is most likely to be affected?

    A   Frontal lobe
    B   Occipital lobe
    C   Parietal lobe
    D   Prefrontal lobe
    E   Temporal lobe

11. Which cognitive function is assessed by verbal frequency?

    A   Executive functions
    B   Language
    C   Memory
    D   Rate of speech
    E   Recall

12. A 35-year-old man was diagnosed with narcissistic personality disorder. Which classification system is used for this diagnosis?

    A   Chinese Classification of Mental Disorders II, revised
    B   DSM-IV
    C   ICD-10

D ICD-9

E Research diagnostic criteria

13. A 29-year-old man was found wandering on the street with some memory loss after his 5-year-old son died suddenly. Which type of memory is most likely to be affected?

    A Episodic memory

    B Implicit memory

    C Procedural memory

    D Semantic memory

    E Working memory

14. Which of the following is a diagnostic criterion for borderline personality disorder in the DSM-IV but not in the ICD-10?

    A Chronic feeling of emptiness

    B Involvement in intense and unstable relationships

    C Recurrent threats or acts of self-harm

    D Transient, stress-related, paranoid ideation

    E Uncertainty about self-image

15. You are seeing a 42-year-old man after a road traffic accident. He was confused and used inappropriate words during the assessment. On the Glasgow coma scale (GCS), what will be the grade of his verbal response?

    A 1

    B 2

    C 3

    D 4

    E 5

16. An 18-year-old woman presented after a road traffic accident. She was confused but cooperated during the assessment. She responded to painful stimulus by withdrawing. On the GCS, what will be the grade of her motor response?

    A 1

    B 2

    C 3

    D 4

    E 5

17. A 45-year-old man with stroke presented with an inability to name the right or left side of his body. In addition, he had writing difficulty, calculation difficulty and speech abnormalities. When he was asked to name his fingers, he could not. Where is the lesion likely to be located in the brain?

    A Frontal lobe

    B Left parietal lobe

    C Left temporal lobe

    D Right parietal lobe

    E Right temporal lobe

18. Which of the following statements about working memory is correct?

    A For the new, long-term, memory process to happen one should have intact working memory

    B It has an unlimited capacity

    C It is analogous to recall after a few minutes

    D It is best tested with the digit-span task

    E Working memory is dependent on long-term memory

19. Which of the following is an example of priming?

    A   Episodic memory
    B   Implicit memory
    C   Semantic memory
    D   Spatial memory
    E   Visual memory

20. A 39-year-old woman presented with symptoms and signs suggestive of generalised anxiety disorder. What should be the minimum duration of these symptoms according to the ICD-10 diagnostic category of generalised anxiety disorder?

    A   1 month
    B   2 months
    C   6 months
    D   1 year
    E   2 years

21. A 55-year-old man presented with foot drop after recently having a plaster cast removed from the same lower limb. There was wasting of the lateral muscles of the lower leg, weakness of dorsiflexion and eversion of the ankle. What would you expect to find to confirm the most likely diagnosis?

    A   Absent ankle reflex
    B   Absent knee reflex
    C   Extensor plantar response
    D   Intact ankle reflex
    E   Intact knee reflex

22. You examined a patient's lower limbs and wanted to grade the muscle weakness. On examination you noted that there was some active movement. What grade does this correspond to according to a Medical Research Council grade?

    A   Grade 0
    B   Grade 1
    C   Grade 2
    D   Grade 3
    E   Grade 4

23. A 75-year-old woman with a history of depression presented with urinary infection and cardiac failure. Which of the following would help to assess her semantic memory?

    A   Correct awareness of passage of time
    B   Giving correct address
    C   Giving correct date of birth
    D   Giving correct place of birth
    E   Naming the correct Prime Minister

24. A 45-year-old woman with a history of depression presented with short-term memory problems. Which of the following bedside tests would best assess the patient's short-term verbal memory?

    A   Copying pentagons
    B   Naming date and place of birth
    C   Orientation in time, place and person
    D   Serial sevens test
    E   Three-word recall

25. A 60-year-old man had an established diagnosis of alcohol dependence. He was admitted to a surgical ward following a fracture of his right leg. He developed Wernicke's encephalopathy and now presents with memory difficulties. Which of the following bedside tests will be impaired?

   A Benton's visual perception
   B Copying pentagons
   C Digit span task
   D Serial sevens test
   E Spelling the word 'world' backwards

26. An 80-year-old man was taking a number of medications for multiple physical problems. He has recently developed a chest and urinary infection and presented in a confused state. Which of the following tests is the least useful to support a diagnosis of delirium?

   A Attention and concentration
   B Clock drawing
   C Name and address test
   D Orientation in time, place and person
   E Remote memory test

27. Which of the following statements about persistent delusional disorder according to the ICD-10 is correct?

   A Delusions must be present for a minimum of 3 months for a diagnosis
   B If depressive symptoms are present they invalidate the diagnosis
   C It is associated with the passivity phenomenon
   D It is associated with persistent auditory hallucinations
   E Somatisation is an essential factor in this disorder

28. What technique is used in the statement 'What do you mean when you say that you have a severe sleep problem?'.

   A Clarification
   B Closed questioning
   C Confrontation
   D Eliciting precision
   E Facilitation

29. An alcohol-dependent patient was examined on admission and his case was handed over to you. Your colleague reported that he had noticed 'cerebellar signs'. Which of the following is of little value as a localising sign?

   A Dysarthria
   B Dysdiadochokinesis
   C Dysmetria
   D Hypotonia
   E Titubation

30. What technique is used in the statement: 'You seem quite upset when you discuss about your son?'

   A Empathy
   B Interpretation
   C Recapitulation
   D Reflection
   E Respectful statement

31. You ask a 70-year-old man who had a stroke recently: 'What did you have for breakfast?' He replied 'cornflakes'. When subsequently asked 'Which medication did you have last night?' and 'How are you?', he again replied 'cornflakes' to both questions. The patient's wife asked what the name for this was so that she could look it up on the internet. What is your response?

     A   Echolalia
     B   Echopraxia
     C   Negativism
     D   Paragrammatism
     E   Perseveration

32. Which of the following statements about anorexia nervosa is correct?

     A   A normal body weight with a distorted body image is pathognomonic of anorexia nervosa
     B   Concordance rates for monozygotic twins are higher than for dizygotic twins
     C   It is less common in enmeshed families
     D   It tends to occur more frequently in lower social classes than in higher social classes
     E   Women with anorexia are more likely to have a history of childhood sexual abuse compared with depressed women

33. Which of the following is a characteristic feature of post-traumatic stress disorder (PTSD)?

     A   A reduced startle reaction is present
     B   It is associated with hypersomnia
     C   Night terrors occur in PTSD
     D   PTSD symptoms usually begin within 6 months of the perceived trauma
     E   Specific EEG changes occur in PTSD

34. Which of the following statements about the Clifton assessment procedures for elderly people is correct?

     A   It does not distinguish between organic and non-organic conditions in elderly people
     B   It has a behaviour rating scale with two subscales
     C   It is a brief measure of psychological functioning, including the level of disability and the need for care in elderly people
     D   The whole assessment is designed to be completed by nurses
     E   The whole assessment is designed to be completed by patients

35. How many axes are there in the DSM-IV?

     A   1
     B   2
     C   3
     D   4
     E   5

36. A 35-year-old lesbian was referred to the outpatient clinic with a 4-month history of low mood, particularly in the morning, difficulty sleeping, poor appetite, weight loss and poor concentration. Which of the following statements about her psychiatric history and prognosis is correct compared with a heterosexual female?

     A   A higher risk of suicide
     B   Less likely to be psychologically distressed
     C   Less likely to have alcohol problems
     D   More likely to have self-harmed
     E   Poorer response to antidepressants

37. Which of the following statements about relapse in schizophrenia is correct?

A   It can be prevented by stress management techniques after the onset of early warning signs
B   It can be successfully treated by intense psychotherapy
C   It can be prevented by intermittent use of medication alone
D   It increases the risk of residual symptoms and social disability after each episode
E   It is not affected by the patient's reaction to the early symptoms

38. Which of the following statements about the significance of deafness and visual impairment is correct?

A   The presence of the two symptoms means that psychotherapeutic approaches are not possible
B   The two symptoms are common in people with learning disabilities
C   They are more often assessed and treated in older adults
D   They multiply rather than add their effect on a person's life
E   They rarely coexist in the adult populations

39. A 42-year-old man was assessed by a liaison psychiatry nurse who thought that he had a somatisation disorder. How long should his symptoms persist before a diagnosis can be made according to the ICD-10?

A   4 months
B   6 months
C   12 months
D   18 months
E   24 months

40. Which of the following statements about the risk of developing Alzheimer's disease (AD) is correct?

A   ApoEε3 is associated with a higher risk of AD
B   Hormone replacement therapy reduces the chance of developing AD
C   Hypertension increases the risk of AD
D   Male sex is a risk factor for developing AD
E   More educated people are at increased risk of AD

41. According to the Terr classification of childhood trauma, which of the following is a type 1 trauma symptom?

A   Cognitive reappraisal
B   Denial
C   Psychic numbing
D   Rage/Self-harm
E   Self-hypnosis

42. An 84-year-old man with a history of falls was brought to the clinic because of recent deterioration in his self-care. He appeared malnourished, confused and somewhat unkempt. It was evident that there was a significant but mild cognitive impairment. What is the most likely diagnosis?

A   Alzheimer's disease
B   Chronic subdural haematoma
C   Multi-infarct dementia
D   Normal pressure hydrocephalus
E   Pick's disease

43. Which of the following is an ICD-10 criterion for anxious (avoidant) personality disorder?

     A   A limited capacity to make everyday decisions
     B   A preoccupation with fears of being left to care for oneself
     C   Excessive preoccupation with being criticised or rejected in social situations
     D   Shallow and labile affectivity
     E   Willingness to get involved with people because of fear or criticism

44. A 22-year-old woman of Asian background was admitted onto the ward. She experienced low mood with suicidal ideation and had attempted to harm herself recently. She confined herself to her bed space. She was noticed to be shy, with low self-esteem and confidence issues. At other times, she was animated while talking to her family. At times, she appeared to be very assertive in her demeanour. She did not respond when addressed by her name and gave a different name. She was also noticed to be acting very childishly, i.e. standing on the sofa and talking in a child-like manner on a few occasions. Her family views this as possession by a demon and they had previously taken her to religious gurus for exorcism. What is the most likely diagnosis?

     A   Borderline personality disorder
     B   Depressive episode
     C   Dissociative disorder
     D   Possession disorder
     E   Schizophrenia

45. A 21-year-old woman was assessed by the junior doctor in the emergency department. She had been evicted from her property where she had lived for 5 years. Previously she had problems with retaining employment and sustaining interpersonal relationships. Her mood was labile at presentation to the emergency department. She expressed strong feelings of rejection, abandonment and paranoia, self-harm and had an unstable sense of self. What is the most likely diagnosis?

     A   Bipolar affective disorder
     B   Borderline personality disorder
     C   Depressive disorder
     D   Dissocial personality disorder
     E   Eating disorder

46. Which of the following characterises type I schizophrenia?

     A   Evidence of dopamine overactivity
     B   Insidious onset
     C   Negative symptoms
     D   Poor response to antipsychotics
     E   Structural brain damage

47. A 28-year-old man presented with a few weeks history of elated mood, increased energy, persecutory ideas and auditory hallucinations. He thinks that he can save the world with his knowledge but aliens are interfering with his thoughts and control him. What is the most likely diagnosis?

     A   Delusional disorder
     B   Mania with psychotic symptoms
     C   Paranoid schizophrenia
     D   Schizoaffective disorder
     E   Schizotypal disorder

48. A 21-year-old woman with an acute first psychotic episode was started on olanzapine 15 mg at night. After 10 days, she developed rigidity, pyrexia and autonomic instability. What is the most likely cause?

     A   Acute dystonia

    B   Encephalitis
    C   Malignant catatonia
    D   Malignant hyperthermia
    E   Neuroleptic malignant syndrome

49. Which of the following disorders is included in the ICD-10 but not in the DSM-IV?

    A   Agoraphobia
    B   Generalised anxiety disorder
    C   Mixed anxiety and depressive disorder
    D   Panic disorder
    E   Social phobia

50. Which of the following statements is correct when comparing the ICD-10 with the DSM-IV?

    A   Both originated from the World Health Organization
    B   The duration for diagnosing schizophrenia is different
    C   The social consequences are included in both systems
    D   The terms 'neurotic' and 'neurasthenia' are not used in the DSM-IV
    E   They do not complement each other

51. Which of the following is included in the DSM-IV but not in the ICD-10?

    A   Dependent personality disorder
    B   Histrionic personality disorder
    C   Narcissistic personality disorder
    D   Paranoid personality disorder
    E   Schizoid personality disorder

52. Which of the following disorders is classified as a personality disorder with the same name and under the same personality disorder category for both the ICD-10 and the DSM-IV?

    A   Anankastic personality disorder
    B   Anxious personality disorder
    C   Dissocial personality disorder
    D   Schizoid personality disorder
    E   Schizotypal personality disorder

53. What does the the ICD-10 multiaxial axis I consist of when compared with the DSM-IV?

    A   DSM-IV first axis
    B   DSM-IV second axis
    C   DSM-IV third axis
    D   DSM-IV fourth axis
    E   DSM-IV – first three axes

54. In the ICD-10, which category describes Ganser's syndrome?

    A   Dissociative (conversion) disorder
    B   Other anxiety disorder
    C   Other neurotic disorder
    D   Reaction to severe stress and adjustment disorders
    E   Somatoform disorder

55. On conducting fundoscopy, you noted that a patient's optic disc appeared pale and swollen. Which of the following conditions can be excluded from the differential diagnosis?

    A   Optic neuritis
    B   Severe anaemia

C   Syphilis
D   Syringomyelia
E   Vitamin B_{12} deficiency

56. Which of the following statements about sodium valproate is correct?

A   Of manic patients 20% respond to valproate in the acute phase
B   Risk of fetal malformations is 4%
C   Sodium valproate causes hypoammonaemia
D   Sodium valproate can be displaced by highly protein-bound drugs
E   Sodium valproate has a simple pharmacokinetic profile

57. Which of the following statements about the mechanism of action of antipsychotic drugs is correct?

A   Amisulpride is a potent $5\text{-}HT_2:D_2$ antagonist
B   Clozapine binds strongly to D_2- but not D_1-receptors while having affinity for D_4-, $5\text{-}HT_2$, $5\text{-}HT_3$, α_1- and α_2-adrenergic, acetylcholine M_1- and H_1-receptors
C   Haloperidol is a potent D_3-receptor blocker
D   Quetiapine has a low affinity for D_1-, D_2- and $5\text{-}HT_2$- receptors and moderate affinity for adrenergic α_1- and α_2-receptors
E   Sulpiride has a dose-related selectivity for postsynaptic D_4- and presynaptic D_2-receptors

58. Which of the following statements describes the most likely situation in which high-dose antipsychotic drugs can be prescribed in patients with schizophrenia?

A   Adjunctive drugs such as antidepressants or mood stabilisers are indicated
B   Compliance with prescribed drugs is doubtful
C   Insufficient time has been allowed for a response
D   Psychological approaches have failed or are inappropriate and the patient remains symptomatic
E   Two different atypical antipsychotic drugs were prescribed

59. What is the mode of action of buspirone?

A   Partial D_2-receptor agonism
B   Partial $5\text{-}HT_{2C}$-receptor antagonism
C   Serotonin partial $5\text{-}HT_{1A}$-receptor agonism
D   Serotonin $5\text{-}HT_{2B}$-receptor antagonism
E   Serotonin $5\text{-}HT_{2C}$-receptor partial agonism

60. Which of the following statements about sleep is correct?

A   As the day progresses, the circadian wake drive increases and homeostatic sleep decreases, until a tipping point is reached, and the ventrolateral preoptic sleep promoter is triggered to release γ-aminobutyric acid in the tuberomammillary nucleus, which increases wakefulness
B   Homeostatic sleep drive increases with a longer period of sleep and decreases with a period in the awake state
C   Sleep consists of multiple phases which recur in a cyclical manner known as the ultradian cycle
D   The diminishing of the circadian wake drive is the result of input to the suprachiasmic nucleus
E   There is a single process regulating sleep

61. Which of the following statements about the possibility of novel glutamergic treatments in schizophrenia is correct?

A   Free radicals are generated in the neurodegenerative processes of inhibito-toxcity

    B   Free radicals such as lazaroids are so named because of the putative properties of raising degenerating neurons

    C   *N*-Methyl-D-aspartate (NMDA) antagonists can potentially block inhibittoxic transmission and exert neuroprotective actions in patients with late-onset schizophrenia

    D   The hypoactivation of NMDA antagonists contributes to the pathophysiology of positive and cognitive symptoms in patients with early onset schizophrenia

    E   As schizophrenia is linked to hyperactive NMDA receptors, agonists at the glycine co-agonist site boost glutamate neurotransmission at NMDA receptors

62. Which of the following statements about drug interactions is correct?

    A   An example of drug interaction is co-administration of carbidopa and levodopa

    B   Drug interactions should be avoided due to poor or unexpected outcomes

    C   Pharmaceutical interactions occur when there is a physicochemical interaction of four compounds in a solution

    D   Pharmacokinetic interactions occur when one drug interferes with the disposition of another only during absorption

    E   Pharmacodynamic interactions occur when two drugs interact at three different sites of action

63. What is the mechanism of action of mirtazapine?

    A   Noradrenergic reuptake inhibitor

    B   Noradrenergic and specific serotoninergic antagonism

    C   Serotoninergic antagonist reuptake inhibitor

    D   Serotonin and noradrenaline reuptake inhibitor

    E   Serotonin selective reuptake inhibitor

64. Dangerous drug interactions can occur between decongestants and drugs that boost sympathomimetic amines such as monoamine oxidase (MAO) inhibitors. Which of the following statements is correct?

    A   Agents that simulate α_1-postsynaptic vascular receptors can be combined with MAO inhibitors for higher effect

    B   Decongestants used together with MAO inhibitors can increase blood pressure

    C   MAO inhibitors can themselves cause hypertension in some patients

    D   MAO inhibitors given on their own do not potentiate noradrenaline

    E   Stimulants, when combined with MAO inhibitors, are safe

65. You are preparing for a lecture for medical students on lithium. Which of the following information should you include in your presentation?

    A   Action of lithium on antidepressants can be considered a form of triaminergic modulation

    B   Action at other sites of signal transduction does not cascade for neurotransmitters down to mood stabilisers

    C   Lithium acts on the enzyme cytochrome P450 (CYP450)

    D   Lithium can decrease the actions of monoamines

    E   The mechanism of action of lithium has been firmly established

66. Which of the following statements is recommended by the National Institute for Health and Care Excellence (NICE) for the long-term management of bipolar affective disorder?

    A   Antipsychotic depot injections should be considered for routine use in these patients

    B   Carbamazepine should be considered as a first-line drug for long-term management

    C   Combination of lithium and sodium valproate should be considered as a first-line treatment for rapidly cycling bipolar affective disorder

    D   Long-term drug treatment should be considered for bipolar I patients with four or more acute episodes

    E   Long-term use of tricyclic antidepressants is recommended to reduce relapse rates of depression

67. According to Erikson's stages of psychosocial development, parenting is an important focus. Which of the following stages is most likely to be involved?

    A   Generativity versus stagnation
    B   Identity versus role confusion
    C   Industry versus inferiority
    D   Intimacy versus isolation
    E   Trust versus mistrust

68. Which is the last stage of psychosocial development as described by Erikson?

    A   Autonomy versus shame and doubt
    B   Generativity versus stagnation
    C   Industry versus inferiority
    D   Integrity versus despair
    E   Intimacy versus isolation

69. Which of the following is considered a part of the collective unconscious?

    A   Archetypes
    B   Defence mechanisms
    C   Ego
    D   Id
    E   Super-ego

70. According to Freud's psychic apparatus, which of the following is concerned with mediating between basic desires and the judicial part of punishment?

    A   Collective unconscious
    B   Dreams
    C   Ego
    D   Id
    E   Super-ego

71. Which of the following terms was first used by Thomas and Chess to refer to the harmonious interactions between a mother and her child?

    A   Attachment
    B   Good-enough mothering
    C   Goodness of fit
    D   Imprinting
    E   Temperament

72. What are phonemes referred to as?

    A   Meaning conveyed by words and sentences
    B   Meaningful part of language
    C   Smallest unit of sound that makes up words
    D   The conventions about combining words according to grammatical rules
    E   The conversational use of language in real social situations

73. A girl starts to realise that she is a girl, which is different from being a boy. How old is she?

    A   2–3 years
    B   3–4 months
    C   4–5 years
    D   6 months to 1 year
    E   7 years

74. Which of the following is the most appropriate combination of fears and corresponding ages?

    A   Fear of loud noises: 7–12 months

    B   Fear of animals: 2–3 years

    C   Fear of bodily injury: 5–8 years

    D   Fear of strangers: birth to 6 months

    E   Fear of disasters: adolescence

75. Which of the following statements about developmental theories is correct?

    A   According to Sigmund Freud, children show interest in their peers in the phallic stage of psychosexual development

    B   A child's ability to view the world from an other's point of view represents the preoperational stage of Jean Piaget

    C   A child who obeys the rules laid down by teachers has reached preconventional stage 1of Jean Piaget's theory

    D   A child has a fear of punishment and guilt which represents Erik Erikson's autonomy vs shame stage

    E   A child shows a gradual increase in interest in the environment and practises exploration; this represents Margaret Mahler's differentiation stage

76. Early life experiences can have a considerable impact on future human deviant or maladaptive behaviour. Which of the following statements about early life experiences is correct?

    A   Psychodynamic psychiatrists rely on current data

    B   Some affection-deprived children are capable of forming attachments

    C   Successful adults usually come from toxic homes

    D   Sigmund Freud postulated a unitary sequence of emotional development

    E   The deviant or maladaptive behaviour is resistant to behavioural treatment approaches

77. Which of the following statements regarding social deprivation in non-human primates is correct?

    A   In total isolation, female primate is able to nurture the young unlike their male partners

    B   Mother only reared primates are terrified of their mother

    C   Peer only reared primates are clingy and timid in their reactions with others

    D   The separation after bonding leads to stereotyped behaviour

    E   There is an initial protest that changes to despair in partially isolated primates

78. A group of football supporters were attacked by a mob of rival supporters after a humiliating defeat of their team. They all became the 'enemy' and even innocent bystanders were attacked. Which of the following social determinants describes this behaviour?

    A   Anonymity

    B   Convergence

    C   Impersonality

    D   Social contagion

    E   Suggestibility

79. What type of message would be the most persuasive communication for the more intelligent recipient?

    A   Explicit messages

    B   High-fear messages

    C   Message repetition

    D   One-sided presentations

    E   Two-sided presentations

80. Which of the following experiments demonstrated the power of conformity?

     A   Asch experiment
     B   Leon Festinger's cognitive dissonance experiment
     C   Milgram's experiment
     D   Muzafer Sherif's robbers cave experiment
     E   Stanford prison experiment

81. A 20-year-old unemployed man has been smoking cannabis for 4–5 years. He did not see this as a problem and said that he used it to relax him and get on with his life. He believed that his parents' worries were excessive. Which of Prochaska and DiClemente's stages of change is reflected here?

     A   Preaction
     B   Precontemplation
     C   Predecision
     D   Pre-evaluation
     E   Premotivation

82. A 41-year-old woman completed her alcohol detoxification at home 6 months ago and has been abstinent since then. Which of Prochaska and DiClemente's stages of change is reflected here?

     A   Action
     B   Contemplation
     C   Decision
     D   Maintenance
     E   Relapse prevention

83. Which of the following therapies works on the basis that the current problems in the family originate from past experiences of individual members?

     A   Cognitive–behavioural therapy
     B   Couples therapy
     C   Flooding
     D   Psychodynamic therapy
     E   Systemic family therapy

84. In psychodynamic psychotherapy, exploration of transference, countertransference and resistance is discussed with a supervisor. When does this happen during the therapy?

     A   Closing session
     B   Early session
     C   Initial assessment
     D   Middle session
     E   Post-therapy session

85. A 58-year-old woman was going through a divorce. Her mother had passed away 6 months ago. She became a grandmother recently. She was not coping with life and sought psychological help. Which is the most appropriate therapy for her?

     A   Community therapy
     B   Group psychotherapy
     C   Interpersonal therapy
     D   Supportive psychotherapy
     E   Therapeutic community

86. Which of the following statements about prevention of substance misuse is correct?

     A   Primary prevention aims to prevent the further progression of a condition by identifying and treating cases at an early stage

B   Primary prevention aims at reducing the prevalence of hazardous drinking or hazards of drinking
C   Primary prevention can be achieved by harm reduction
D   Secondary prevention can be achieved by controlling the availability of alcohol and drugs
E   Secondary prevention can be achieved by targeting the whole population

87. Who was a major figure in psychiatry and neurology from 1856 to 1926 and also created the term 'dementia praecox'?

A   Bleuler
B   Hecker
C   Kahlbaum
D   Kraepelin
E   Morel

88. Which French psychiatrist from the eighteenth century used a term to describe deteriorated patients whose illness began in adolescence?

A   Bleuler
B   Hecker
C   Kahlbaum
D   Kraepelin
E   Morel

89. In which year did Jacob Kasanin introduce the term 'schizoaffective disorder'?

A   1928
B   1930
C   1933
D   1935
E   1938

90. A 26-year-old unmarried woman was unaware of her hatred towards her mother. However, she often felt inexplicably resentful towards older women in positions of authority. She could not understand why she had felt like this for several years. Which of the following can explain this situation?

A   Altruism
B   Displacement
C   Idealisation
D   Projection
E   Projective identification

91. A 49-year-old single man had been devoted to his mother but was cold and distant with his 80-year-old father. He was unaware of his sexual interest in his mother for many years and his death wish for his father. Which of the following can explain this situation?

A   Rationalisation
B   Reaction formation
C   Regression
D   Repression
E   Splitting

92. A 55-year-old male lawyer wished for his child to be a lawyer too, but unfortunately the child died in a car accident. Since the child's death, the lawyer has started to offer free legal advice to students. Which is the most likely defence mechanism?

A   Acting out

B   Altruism
C   Humour
D   Reaction formation
E   Sublimation

93. A 29-year-old woman had an affair with her neighbour but she accused her husband of cheating on her. What is the most likely phenomenon?

A   Acting out
B   Projection
C   Rationalisation
D   Regression
E   Repression

94. In which category of the DSM-IV is schizotypal disorder classified?

A   Affective disorders
B   Disorders of psychological development
C   Neurotic, stress-related and somatoform disorders
D   Personality disorders
E   Schizophrenia and related disorders

95. A 30-year-old male professional footballer was not able to score an easy goal in a Premier League match. Since then, he has started to think that he was not a good player. Which is the most likely cognitive distortion?

A   Black-and-white thinking
B   Catastrophic thinking
C   Projection
D   Rationalisation
E   Selective abstraction

96. Who was the first person to describe the condition currently known as schizoaffective disorder?

A   Bleuler
B   Cade
C   Deniker
D   Kahlbaum
E   Kasanin

97. Who first described a condition called *folie circulaire*?

A   Celsus
B   Hippocrates
C   Jules Falret
D   Kahlbaum
E   Kraepelin

98. Erikson's stages of human psychosexual development differ from those of Freud in several areas. Which of the following is one such area?

A   Development depends on successful negotiation of stages
B   Erickson's stages have both positive and negative aspects
C   They extend beyond young adulthood
D   The emphasis is on external events
E   They both follow the theory of infantile sexuality

99. With what is Jean-Martin Charcot most credited?

A   Classification of neurology
B   Discovering nerve conduction
C   Mapping the cerebral cortex
D   The existence of neurotransmitters
E   The practice of hypnosis

100. According to Jean Piaget, the semiotic function in children emerges during their cognitive development. In which stage of cognitive development does this happen?

A   Concrete operational stage
B   Formal operations
C   At any stage
D   Preoperational stage
E   Sensorimotor stage

101. Which phenomenon did Margaret Mead describe in her book *Coming of Age in Samoa*?

A   An absence of adolescent turmoil such as competitiveness/aggression
B   The lack of tribal rivalry because they were peace loving
C   The low incidence of suicide among young people in the society
D   The Oedipus complex in Samoan societies
E   The passing rites/rituals of adolescent girls

102. Which of the following in human beings was prompted by the work of the great ethologist Karl Von Frish?

A   Aggressive behaviour in humans
B   Characteristics of human communication systems
C   Human response to stress
D   Patterns of human attachment behaviour
E   Sexual behaviour in humans

103. Which law is made by a legislative process, according to the British judicial system?

A   Civil law
B   Common law
C   Criminal law
D   Negligence
E   Statute law

104. A 45-year-old man was shocked when he looked into the mirror and did not see his reflection. What is this phenomenon called?

A   Hygric hallucination
B   Hypnogogic hallucination
C   Hypnopompic hallucination
D   Negative autoscopic hallucination
E   Pseudo-hallucination

105. A 22-year-old medical student was searching the literature for depression and EEG. She was interested in knowing what changes would be seen in depression. What is the most likely EEG change seen in depression?

A   Decreased rapid eye movement (REM) sleep
B   Decreased slow-wave sleep
C   Increased delta waves
D   Increased slow-wave sleep
E   No change

106. According to Melanie Klein's theory of psychoanalysis what does the paranoid–schizoid position stand for?

    A   Children realise that their mothers have both positive and negative aspects

    B   An infant projects feelings of rage and hatred on to the mother and fears the same feelings from the mother

    C   The infant splits his or her experiences into 'good' and 'bad' elements of the mother and him- or herself

    D   The infant fears attack from the 'bad' mother

    E   The infant has unconscious knowledge of bodily functions

107. Who propagated the person-centred theory of personality and psychotherapy?

    A   Adolf Meyer

    B   Carl Rogers

    C   Harry Stack Sullivan

    D   Jean-Paul Sartre

    E   Otto Rank

108. Which of the following psychotropic drugs has high absorption of moisture when it comes into contact with moist air or humidity?

    A   Carbamazepine

    B   Lamotrigine

    C   Lithium

    D   Risperidone

    E   Sodium valproate

109. Which of the following statements about Carl Jung is correct?

    A   Jung's concept of the 'Anima' referred to the feminine qualities of a man

    B   Jung continued to work on Freud's ideas of infantile sexuality

    C   Jung described the concept of the collective unconscious

    D   Jung described 'persona' as a person's true identity

    E   Jung was influenced by antiquity and ancient Greek mythologies

110. Who was the first person to use the terms 'mania' and 'melancholia' to describe mental illness?

    A   Celsus

    B   Hippocrates

    C   Jules Falret

    D   Kahlbaum

    E   Kraepelin

111. Who is credited as the first people to describe the social origins of depression?

    A   Avison and Robins

    B   Barton

    C   Brown and Harris

    D   Goffman

    E   Maxwell Jones

112. Which of the following does not form one of the criteria for acute intoxication of alcohol in the ICD-10?

    A   Argumentativeness

    B   Intoxication occurring soon after consumption of alcohol

    C   Lability of mood

D   Slurred speech
E   Unsteady gait

113. Which of the following statements about lithium is correct?

    A   Abrupt lithium withdrawal leads to rapid relapse into depression
    B   Concomitant use of angiotensin-converting enzyme inhibitors leads to decreased serum lithium levels
    C   Concomitant use of serotonin selective reuptake inhibitors can lead to the serotonin syndrome
    D   Concomitant use of theophylline leads to decreased serum lithium levels
    E   Furosemide is contraindicated with lithium

114. Who said 'Is there such a thing as mental illness?' and is also known for the antipsychiatry movement?

    A   David Cooper
    B   L Ron Hubbard
    C   Michael Foucault
    D   RD Laing
    E   Thomas Szasz

115. In western Europe, which court has the highest binding power?

    A   Court of appeal
    B   Crown court
    C   European court
    D   High court
    E   Supreme court

116. What is the likelihood of people having a middle-ear infection developing schizophrenia compared with the general population?

    A   0.9 times
    B   1.8 times
    C   3.6 times
    D   4.5 times
    E   5.4 times

Answers: MCQs

1. B Consider taking notes after the assessment has been completed

When seeing an angry or agitated patient, try to keep the following in mind: first of all, ensure your own safety. Consider having a chaperone accompany you and it is advisable to carry a panic alarm. Avoid seating the patient between the interviewer and the door. Do not sit directly opposite the patient and avoid sitting too close so that you do not invade his or her personal space. It is worth considering taking notes after the assessment.

2. C To control an over-talkative patient during the assessment

Closed questions usually elicit a specific answer such as 'yes' or 'no' and are helpful during the course of an interview after open questions. Unstructured interviews are usually employed in dynamically informed practice. A chaperone may be present when a patient is angry or aggressive and a balance of interview styles is used. Silence is helpful when the patient accepts or contemplates something. During an interview with an over-talkative patient, it can be helpful to use closed questions.

3. A Closed question

These are mainly used in the latter part of a psychiatric interview and help in making the differential diagnosis. The answer of a closed question is usually 'yes' or 'no'. Some examples of closed questions are 'Do you feel suicidal?', 'Do you have suicidal thoughts?', 'Do you feel hopeless?' and 'Do you feel helpless?'

4. D Leading question

Questions that lead a patient towards a specific response are called leading questions. They can be of two types. There are positive leading questions and negative leading questions. An example of a positive leading question is 'You were happy at that time?' and a negative leading question is 'You were not happy at that time'?.

5. C Directive question

These are also called imperative questions. This questioning style uses commands, e.g. 'Tell me more about your low mood', 'Tell me more about what had happened on the day that you took the overdose'. Directive questioning style is used in over-talkative patients and in cases where you are required to direct the patient to a particular area and gather more information about it.

6. D Parietal lobe

Constructional abilities are function of the non-dominant parietal lobe. Constructional apraxia is caused by an impaired parietal lobe.

7. E Registration

Orientation is tested by checking the person's awareness of place and date through a series of questions. Registration is tested by first asking the person to name three objects. Then, the person is asked to spell the word 'WORLD' backwards, or the serial sevens test is used to test attention and orientation. Then, asking the person to repeat the names of the three objects tests recall.

8. E True insight

Insight is defined as conscious recognition of one's own condition.

True insight – increased knowledge about self or situation and motivation to use this knowledge to bring about an effective change in behaviour.

Intellectual insight – increased knowledge about self or situation but unable to use this knowledge to bring about an effective change in behaviour.

Action and contemplation – Prochaska and DiClemente's stages of change.

9. D Rorschach's inkblot test

Projective personality tests were developed from an idiographic, psychodynamic perspective, in particular that deeper layers of an individual's personality contain repressed wishes, impulses and desires that are not always accessible via conscious self-report. The two most widely used instruments are Rorschach's inkblot test and the thematic apperception test. Cattell used 16 personality factors expressed as dimensions, e.g. tense versus relaxed, outgoing versus reserved. The Rey–Osterrieth test is used for visual memory.

10. C Parietal lobe

A variety of formal cognitive tests can assess parietal lobe function. These are visual perception, time perception, Raven's Progressive matrices, visual construction (the Rey–Osterrieth Complex Figure, drawing interlocking polygons, clock drawing) and right–left orientation.

11. A Executive functions

An executive function refers to the complex of abilities that allows us to plan, initiate, organise and monitor our thoughts and behaviour. These abilities are located mainly in the frontal lobes and are essential for normal social performance. Verbal fluency, motor sequencing, the go–on–go test and test of abstraction are some of the specific tests for clarifying deficits in frontal lobe function.

12. B DSM-IV only

Narcissistic personality disorder is a diagnostic criterion not available in the ICD-10. It is a diagnosis in the DSM-IV. According to the criteria, the person has a grandiose sense of self-importance; preoccupied with fantasies of unlimited success, he believes that he is special or unique, requires excessive admiration, lacks empathy, and shows arrogant and haughty behaviour.

13. D Loss of semantic memory

This short scenario is about the fugue state, precipitated by his son's death. Semantic memory is affected in the fugue state.

14. D Transient stress-related paranoid ideation

Borderline personality disorder was originally used to describe individuals with instability. In the DSM-IV, there is an additional criterion not mentioned in the ICD-10 – transient paranoia.

15. C 3

Best verbal response on the GCS is scored as follows:

1 = none
2 = incomprehensible sounds
3 = inappropriate words
4 = confused
5 = oriented

16. C 3

Best motor response on the GCS is scored as follows:

1 = none
2 = extending to pain
3 = flexes abnormally (spastic flexion)
4 = withdraws (normal flexion)
5 = localises pain
6 = obeys commands

17. B Left parietal lobe lesion

The clinical scenario suggests Gerstmann's syndrome which is as a result of damage to the left parietal lobe. The main symptoms are agraphia or dysgraphia, acalculia or dyscalculia, finger agnosia and left–right disorientation.

18. D It is best tested with the digit-span task

Previously, it was thought that immediate memory should be intact for new learning. However, now it has been proved that they are parallel. Immediate/working memory has limited capacity. It is best tested with the digit-span task.

19. B Implicit memory

Priming is a type of implicit memory. In priming, exposure to the test stimulus improves the performance of the organism. This might happen even if the organism has no conscious recollection of the event.

20. C 6 months

The symptoms of generalised anxiety disorder consist of prominent tension, worry, apprehension about daily events for a period of 6 months, along with at least four symptoms of autonomic arousal pertaining to the chest and abdomen. It is not part of the subcategory of phobic anxiety disorders.

21. D Intact ankle reflex

This is a case of common peroneal nerve palsy. This nerve is one of the branches of the sciatic nerve and can be compressed by a plaster cast, as in this case. The tibial branch of the sciatic nerve conveys the ankle reflex and, hence, the ankle reflex should remain intact.

22. C Grade 2

Table 5.1 Muscle weakness grading

Muscle weakness grading	
0	No muscle contraction
1	Flicker of contraction
2	Some active movement
3	Active movement against gravity
4	Active movement against resistance
5	Normal power (allowing for age)

23. E Naming the correct Prime Minister

Semantic memory refers to memory for abstract facts such as the name of the current Prime Minister, capital cities. Autobiographical memory refers to memories for events and issues that relate to oneself. It is characterised by a general recall of the event, an interpretation of the event and a recall of a few specific details.

24. E Three-word recall

Three-word recall is a bedside test that can assess short-term memory problems. The patient is given a task to repeat back three words, digits or information immediately without delay. Three to four attempts are permissible. This test is about immediate registration and recall that tests short-term memory.

25. C Digit span task

This is a standard test of short-term memory, the store that holds a limited amount of information for periods of up to 30 seconds. Immediate recall of a name and address may also reflect partly or wholly the operation of short-term memory. Delayed recall of the same name and address tests long-term memory; the store of all information needs to be held for more than 30 seconds.

26. B Clock drawing

In delirium, the patient exhibits impairment of consciousness, attention, concentration and short-term memory. Orientation in time, place and person is also impaired.

27. A Delusions must be present for a minimum of 3 months for a diagnosis

This is a disorder characterised by the development of either a single delusion or a set of related delusions that are usually persistent and sometimes lifelong. There must be no persistent hallucinations in any modality, but there may be transitory or occasional auditory hallucinations that are not in the third person or give a running commentary.

28. A Clarification

Closed questions are geared towards some factual response about which there is little room for debate. Facilitation encourages the patient to continue along a particular line of thought. It helps the interview to flow, establish a rapport and gain patients' confidence.

29. D Hypotonia

Cerebellar signs include:

- Ataxic gait (patient falters towards the side of the lesion)
- Movement is imprecise in force and in distance (dysmetria)
- Rapid alternating movements are clumsy and disorganised (dysdiadochokinesis)
- Titubation (rhythmic tremor of the head in either to-and-fro or rotary movements
- Dysarthria – speech often reported as being scanning or staccato in severe cases
- Intention tremor
- Nystagmus – hypotonia and depression of reflexes are sometime seen but are of little value as localising signs.

30. D Reflection

This refers to when the interviewer repeats what the patient has just said. Interpretation refers to inferences of behaviour or thoughts reached by the interviewer. Recapitulation and summarising allow for clarification for providing a natural break for 'air'. They also allow the interviewer to facilitate the interview by offering approbation for the efforts so far.

31. E Perseveration

This occurs when mental operations persist beyond the point at which they are relevant and thus prevent progress of thinking. It may be verbal or ideational. In the early stages of perseveration, the patient may recognise the difficulty and try to overcome it. Paragrammatism means a speech disorder characterised by faulty grammar or syntactic relationship. Echolalia means compulsive repetition of words spoken by others. Echopraxis means compulsive imitation of actions and echo kinesis means compulsive imitation of movements. Negativism is considered as an accentuation of opposition. It is often used to describe hostility, motivated refusal and failure to cooperate.

32. B Concordance rates for monozygotic twins are higher than for dizygotic twins

The evidence from twin studies suggests that specific genetic factors are more important in anorexia nervosa (AN) than in bulimia nervosa (BN), particularly in restricting (or AN) where concordance rates from monozygotic twins are higher compared with dizygotic twins. Sociodemographic factors such as social class, parental age, family composition and family size are suggested as contributing factors, but none of them has been found consistently across studies.

33. D PTSD symptoms usually begin within 6 months of the perceived trauma

The post-traumatic stress disorder (PTSD) is a delayed and/or protracted response to exceptionally threatening or catastrophic events or situations that usually begin within 6 months of the perceived trauma. Three clusters of symptoms characterise PTSD. They are: (1) intrusive and uncontrollable re-experiencing of aspects of the provoking stressor or trauma; (2) deliberate attempts to avoid remembering or re-living the traumatic experience; and (3) hyperarousal, increased vigilance, exaggerated startle response, irritability, poor concentration and insomnia.

34. C It is a brief measure of psychological functioning, including the level of disability and the need for care in elderly people

Clifton's assessment procedures for the elderly (CAPE) is a brief assessment procedure for elderly patients. It consists of 12 items scored by nurses or other staff who know the patients. It includes orientation, and mental abilities such as counting, reading, writing and repeating the alphabet. Scores derived from CAPE have been shown to have good predictive validity in terms of outcome at follow-up and in the distinction between functional and organic mental disorders in elderly people.

35. E 5

There are five axes in the DSM-IV classification:

Axis I: clinical disorders
Axis II: personality disorders and mental retardation (learning disability)
Axis III: General medical conditions
Axis IV: psychosocial and environment problems
Axis V: global assessment of functioning

36. D More likely to have self-harmed

Studies examining sexual orientation and mental health found a higher prevalence of anxiety, depression and substance misuse, suicidal ideation and attempts in homosexual compared with heterosexual populations. It is postulated that stresses due to stigmatisation and exposure to discriminatory behaviour lead to higher rates of mental disorders in homosexuals. Between 20% and 42% of homosexual adolescents attempt suicide, the attempts being generally more serious and more often fatal than those of their heterosexual counterparts.

37. D It increases the risk of residual symptoms and social disability after each episode

The outcome of schizophrenia, as Kraepelin himself would eventually realise, is very variable, regardless of how the syndrome is defined. Some symptoms resolve completely with or without treatment and some never resolve. Some patients recover after each episode. Others achieve an incomplete recovery. Some patients experience a persistent defect state that does not improve or tends indeed to deteriorate with successive relapses. There is consistent evidence that reducing or stopping antipsychotic medication, even after a prolonged period of maintenance and well-being, is a risk for relapse.

38. B The two symptoms are common in people with learning disabilities

Sensory information, e.g. deafness, has been shown to be associated with 25–40% of patients with old age schizophrenia. Visual impairment is less relevant. These impairments are not well assessed in the older adults.

39. E 24 months

The features of somatisation disorder (Briquet's syndrome) are multiple, recurrent and frequently changing symptoms, spread over the minimum duration of 2 years. The symptoms emanate from multiple systems of the body. The diagnosis is supported by negative investigations and several unremarkable exploratory operations might have to be performed.

40. C Hypertension increases the risk of AD

There is now increasing evidence of a positive association between AD and vascular risk factors such as type 1 diabetes, hypertension and smoking. Women are at an increased risk of AD, possibly due to hormonal factors. Poor education, especially in males, increases the risk of AD. Mutations in presenilin genes (*PS-1* located on chromosome 14 and *PS-2* located on chromosome 1) are inherited as an autosocial dominant pattern and are fully penetrant. Apolipoprotein (ApoE) ε4 allele is a 'dose-dependent' risk factor for late-onset AD. It is associated with a much higher risk than the ApoEε3 allele. ApoEε2 acts as a protective factor for developing AD.

41. A Cognitive reappraisal

According to the Terr classification of childhood trauma, type 1 trauma is most common and occurs after an acute single traumatic event. The symptoms of type 1 trauma are fully detailed memories, cognitive reappraisal and misperceptions. Type 2 trauma is due to repeated exposure to extreme external events and the symptoms are denial and psychic numbing, self-hypnosis, depersonalisation, dissociation, rage, self-harm and/or extreme passivity.

42. B Chronic subdural haematoma

Subdural haematomas are accumulations of blood and blood products in the space between the fibrous dura matter and the arachnoid membrane, which encloses the brain. Acute subdural haematomas are diagnosed close to the time of trauma. The symptoms include headaches, depressed level of consciousness and focal neurological signs. Chronic subdural haematomas give rise to more gradually evolving features, sometimes resulting in confusion and dementia. Marked variability of mental state is often a clue to diagnosis.

43. C Excessive preoccupation with being criticised or rejected in social situations

Patients with anxious (avoidant) personality disorder are preoccupied with the idea that they will be criticised, disapproved of or rejected in social situations. As a result of this fear and preoccupation, patients avoid engaging in a relationship or social situation. Patients with this disorder have feelings of being inadequate and have a poor self-esteem. They think that they are inferior to others. They are highly self-conscious, shy and timid, and have a strong sense of feeling lonely. They are highly sensitive to rejection and criticism by others.

44. C Dissociative disorder

There are several types: dissociative identity disorder previously known as multiple personality disorder is one type. There are two or more distinct personalities existing within one person with this disorder. The person has distinct memories and behaviour, and at certain times one of the personalities takes over. There is inconsistency in the history with a denial of apparent incidents. In possession disorder, the person him- or herself thinks he or she is being possessed by a spirit.

45. B Borderline personality disorder

Those with borderline personality disorder (BPD) suffer from affective instability, unstable relationships, impulsivity, chronic emptiness, unstable sense of self, suicidal behaviours, difficulty controlling anger and efforts to avoid abandonment. Nowadays there is a barrage of referrals for labelling people with a diagnosis of bipolar affective disorder, whereas in reality they meet the diagnosis of BPD. Individuals with bipolar affective disorder experience symptoms of mood instability with decreased sleep and disinhibition in bouts, which can be frequent or infrequent. Contrary to this, borderline personality disorder, in which the symptoms are persistent on a daily basis, at times, and triggers can be trivial day-to-day incidents.

46. A Evidence of dopamine overactivity

Professor Tim Crow, a British psychiatrist, has described two syndromes of schizophrenia. The characteristics of these syndromes are as shown in **Table 5.2**.

Table 5.2 Type I and type II schizophrenia

	Type I	Type II
Onset	Acute	Insidious
Main symptoms	Positive	Negative
Social functioning	Preserved during remission	Poor
Response to antipsychotic	Good	Poor
Dopamine overactivity	Evidence present	Evidence absent
Structural brain change	Not present	Present, mainly ventricular enlargement

47. D Schizoaffective disorder

- **Schizoaffective disorder:** schizophrenic and affective symptoms occur simultaneously or at least within a few days of each other in the same episode of illness. The episode does not meet the criteria for schizophrenia or affective disorder alone.
- **Delusional disorder:** this can be safely ruled out because there is no history of schizophrenic symptoms and no or occasional auditory hallucinations.
- **Mania with psychotic symptoms:** there will be predominantly severe manic symptoms and psychotic symptoms will follow the affective symptoms.
- **Paranoid schizophrenia:** there will not have been simultaneous affective symptoms
- **Schizotypal disorder:** this does not have any dominant or typical disturbance such as schizophrenia or affective disorder. Its course is similar to a personality disorder. Also, the typical features should be present for at least 2 years.

48. E Neuroleptic malignant syndrome

The following are differential diagnoses of neuroleptic malignant syndrome (NMS):

- **Neuroleptic malignant syndrome:** according to the DSM-IV, NMS is characterised by muscle rigidity and an elevated temperature associated with the administration of an antipsychotic medication. Two or more symptoms of autonomic instability need to be present, and blood investigations should be instigated. There is an absence of infection, general medical condition or substance use that may result in a similar condition. It is estimated to occur in 0.2–1% of patients treated with dopamine-blocking agents. It is also known to occur in other neurological disorders (e.g. Wilson's disease, Parkinson's disease treated with dopamine-blocking agents).

It may also occur in patients treated with dopamine antagonists given for nausea (e.g. metoclopramide, prochlorperazine).

- **Encephalitis:** this may present with a viral prodrome, meningeal signs, other neurological signs, seizures, and imaging and cerebrospinal fluid abnormalities.
- **Acute dystonia:** this is usually not associated with pyrexia and autonomic instability.
- **Malignant catatonia:** idiopathic malignant catatonia is due to advanced stages of psychosis and may be difficult to differentiate from NMS, which is also thought to be an iatrogenic malignant catatonia.
- **Malignant hyperthermia:** this occurs after an administration of some general anaesthetic agents, such as potent volatile agents, e.g. halothane, suxamethonium.

49. C Mixed anxiety and depressive disorder

This is included in the ICD-10 but not in the DSM-IV. The other options are included in both the ICD-10 and the DSM-IV.

50. B Duration for diagnosing schizophrenia is different

Both the classification systems, ICD-10 and DSM-IV, are complementary to each other. In the ICD-10, the guidelines and criteria do not include the social consequences of the disorder. It requires 1 month of symptoms for a diagnosis of schizophrenia, but according to the DSM-IV it requires 6 months including prodromal symptoms. The term 'neurotic' or 'neurasthenia' is not used in the DSM-IV.

51. C Narcissistic personality disorder

The narcissistic and passive–aggressive personality disorder present in the DSM-IV but not in the ICD-10. The dependent, histrionic, paranoid and schizoid personality disorders are present in both the ICD-10 and the DSM-IV.

52. D Schizoid personality disorder

The schizoid personality is present in both the ICD-10 and the DSM-IV.

- **Anankastic:** obsessive–compulsive personality disorder
- **Anxious:** avoidant disorder
- **Dissocial:** antisocial disorder
- **Schizoid:** schizoid disorder

Schizotypal disorder is classified with schizophrenia in the ICD-10 but in the DSM-IV it is classified as a personality disorder.

53. E DSM-IV – first three axes

The ICD-10 axis includes the first three DSM-IV axes which are psychiatric disorders, personality disorders, mental retardation (learning disabilities) and medical illness. Axis II assesses the disability resulting from the axis-I and it uses a short disability assessment schedule. Axis IV corresponds to axis IV of the DSM-IV.

54. A Dissociative (conversion) disorder

In Ganser's syndrome, a patient gives approximate answers to a question. He also has psychosomatic symptoms, abnormal perceptions such as hallucinations and clouding of consciousness.

55. D Syringomyelia

There are many causes of optic nerve lesions, which include the causes of optic neuritis.

Syringomyelia is most unlikely to be the cause because this is a fluid-filled cavity within the spinal cord and presents with dissociated sensory loss, loss of upper limb reflexes, wasting of the small muscles of the hand and forearm, spastic paraparesis and neuropathic joints. If it extends into the brain stem (syringobulbia); Horner's syndrome can be a feature.

All other options can result in a pale and swollen optic disc.

56. D Sodium valproate can be displaced by highly protein-bound drugs

Approximately 50% of manic patients respond to valproate in the acute phase. Sodium valproate causes hyperammonaemia and gastric irritation which can lead to intense nausea. The risk of fetal malformation is 7.2%, mainly due to neural tube defects.

Valproate is highly protein bound. Other drugs that are also highly protein bound, such as aspirin, can displace valproate from albumin, leading to toxicity.

Valproate has a complex pharmacokinetic profile following a three-compartment model and showing protein-bound saturation.

57. D Quetiapine has a low affinity for D_1-, D_2- and 5-HT$_2$ receptors and moderate affinity for adrenergic α_1- and α_2-receptors

Haloperidol is a potent D_2-receptor blocker. Clozapine binds weakly to D_1- and D_2-receptors while having affinity for D_4-, 5-HT$_2$, 5-HT$_3$, α_1- and α_2-adrenergic, acetylcholine M_1- and H_1-receptors. Sulpiride has dose-related selectivity for postsynaptic D_2- and presynaptic D_4-receptors. Risperidone is a potent 5-HT$_2$:D_2-receptor antagonist. Amisulpride selectively blocks presynaptic dopamine receptors.

58. D Psychological approaches have failed or are inappropriate and the patient remains symptomatic

Before prescribing high doses, ensure that sufficient time is allowed for a response. At least two different antipsychotics should have been tried, one of which is an atypical antipsychotic drug. There should be no doubt about compliance. Adjunctive medications such as antidepressants or mood stabilisers are not indicated.

59. C Serotonin partial 5-HT$_{1A}$-receptor agonism

Agomelatine has both serotonin partial 5-HT$_{2C}$- and 5-HT$_{2B}$-receptor antagonistic properties. Aripiprazole is a partial D_2-receptor agonist.

60. C Sleep consists of multiple phases which recur in a cyclical manner, known as the ultradian cycle

Several processes regulate sleep. The circadian wake drive is the result of input to the suprachiasmic nucleus. Homeostatic sleep drive decreases the longer one is asleep, and increases the longer one is awake. As the day progresses, circadian wake drive decreases and homeostatic sleep increases until a tipping point is reached and the ventrolateral sleep preoptic is triggered to release γ-aminobutyric acid in the tuberomammilary nucleus and inhibit wakefulness.

61. B Free radicals such as lazaroids are so named because of the putative properties of raising degenerating neurons

N-Methyl-D-aspartate (NMDA) antagonists could potentially block excitotoxic transmission and exert neuroprotective actions in early schizophrenia. Hypoactivation of NMDA antagonists' contributes to the pathophysiology of positive and cognitive symptoms in late schizophrenia. Free radicals are generated in the neurodegenerative processes of excitotoxicity. So as the answer says, free radicals such as lazaroids are so named because of the putative properties of raising degenerating neurons. As schizophrenia may be linked to hypoactive NMDA receptors, agonists at the glycine co-agonist site may boost glutamate neurotransmission at NMDA receptors, in a manner sufficient to reduce hypoactivity and enhance NMDA currents.

62. A An example of drug interaction is co-administration of carbidopa with levodopa

Drug interactions do not necessarily need to be avoided. Pharmaceutical interactions occur when there is a physicochemical interaction between two compounds in solution. Pharmacokinetic interactions occur when one drug interferes with the disposition of another during absorption, distribution and elimination. Pharmacodynamic interactions occur when two drugs interact at the same site of action.

There may be beneficial effects, e.g. co-administration of carbidopa and levodopa, which allows levodopa to be available in the brain without being metabolised.

63. B Noradrenergic and specific serotoninergic antagonism

The mechanism of action of antidepressants listed are:

Noradrenergic and specific serotoninergic antagonism: mirtazapine
Serotonergic antagonist reuptake inhibitor: trazadone
Serotonin selective reuptake inhibitors: fluoxetine, citalopram, sertraline, paroxetine, fluvoxamine
Noradrenergic reuptake inhibitor: reboxetine
Serotonin and noradrenaline reuptake inhibitor: venlafaxine

64. B Decongestants used with MAO inhibitors can increase blood pressure

Agents that simulate α_1- postsynaptic vascular receptors should be avoided with MAO inhibitors. MAO inhibitors by themselves can cause orthostatic hypotension; they potentiate noradrenaline but this is not sufficient to cause hypertension. In fact, if anything, MAO inhibitors are likely to cause hypotension. The problem comes only when MAO inhibitors are combined with decongestants or other drugs/substances such as amphetamine that increase noradrenaline. Hence, stimulants such as amphetamines should not be combined with MAO inhibitors.

65. A Actions of lithium on antidepressants can be considered a form of triaminergic modulation

The mechanism of action of lithium is still debated and has not yet been firmly established. This may be because of action on the enzyme glycogen synthetase kinase. Lithium can boost the actions of monoamines by mechanisms that are poorly understood, and actions on other sites of the signal transduction cascade for the neurotransmitters of mood stabilisers.

66. C Combination of lithium and sodium valproate should be considered as a first-line treatment for rapidly cycling bipolar affective disorder

The NICE guidelines offer advice on the long-term management of bipolar affective disorder. They recommend long-term management of bipolar I disorder with two or more acute episodes, and bipolar II disorder with significant functional impairment, high suicide risk and frequent episodes. The guidelines include advice on drug treatment after full recovery from acute eposodes, chronic and recurrent depressive symptoms, rapidly cycling disorders and comorbid anxiety disorders. They also provide advice on promoting a healthy lifestyle, preventing relapse, psychological therapies and psychosocial support. The guide-lines recommend a combination of lithium and valproate for rapidly cycling disorders and serotonin selective reuptake inhibitors in minimal therapeutic doses together with mood stabilisers for treatment of chronic and recurrent depressive symptoms.

67. A Generativity versus stagnation

Erikson has described eight stages of psychosocial development.

Table 5.3 Erik Erikson's stages of psychosocial development	
Stage 1	• 0–1 year: trust versus mistrust
Stage 2	• 1–3 years: autonomy versus shame and guilt
Stage 3	• 3–6 years: initiative versus guilt
Stage 4	• 6–12 years: industry versus inferiority
Stage 5	• 12–18 years: identity versus role confusion
Stage 6	• 20s: intimacy versus isolation
Stage 7	• Late 20s to 50s: generativity versus stagnation
Stage 8	• 50s and beyond: integrity versus despair

68. D Integrity versus despair

Erikson, a student of Freud, accepted the basic theory of early psychosocial development but proposed that development continues across the lifespan, particularly in terms of the developing relationship between the individual and the social system within which they live. He underlined the social context for this final stage of growth. In *Childhood and Society*, he wrote, 'the style of integrity developed by his culture or civilisation thus becomes the "patrimony" of his soul. In such final consolidation, death loses its sting. When the attempt to attain integrity has failed, the individual may become deeply disgusted with external world and contemptuous of persons as well institutions'.

69. A Archetypes

Jung described the collective unconscious which contains latent images of psyche development. There are several types described. The four major types described are:

1. **Persona:** 'mask' is the outward face that we present to the world.
2. **Anima and animus:** unconscious mirror of gender; if we are male our animus is of unconscious female and if we are female our animus is of unconscious male.
3. **The shadow:** contains more of our basic animal nature.
4. **The self:** the 'archetypes of archetypes' which unites and gives rise to oneness.

70. C Ego

According to Freud the psychic apparatus is made up of three parts:

1. **Id:** basic and innate desires
2. **Ego:** executive part that balances the id and super-ego
3. **Super-ego:** concerned with punishment; the moral part.

71. C Goodness of fit

Goodness of fit was introduced by Thomas and Chess and it results when the opportunities, demands and expectations of the parents and others are in consonance with the child's temperament and other abilities. Winnicott called a mother who was attuned to the mental state and emotional needs of an infant a 'good-enough mother'. Attachment is explained by John Bowlby as a dyadic affective tie between the mother and the infant. Imprinting is a term coined by Lorenz to describe the distinctive process by which young newly hatched birds learn the characteristics of their mothers and therefore their species. Thomas and Chess describe temperament as a phenomenological term that describes behavioural tendencies that have no etiological implications, and also as a characteristic that is open to environmental influences and developmental maturation.

72. C Smallest unit of sound that makes up words

A refers to morphemes, and words are made up of one or more morphemes. B refers to semantics. Pragmatics is the conversational use of language in real social situations and different contexts. E is the description of syntax.

73. A 2–3 years

Gender identity is a child's understanding of whether they are male or female. It develops around 2–3 years of age, followed by gender stability (permanence of gender identity) by about 4 years of age. Gender constancy (gender identity unalterable by change in appearance) appears around 6 years of age.

74. B Fear of animals: 2–3 years

Normal fears in childhood:

0–6 months → fear of fall, loud noises, loss of support
7–12 months → fear of height, depth, strangers
1 year → fear of separation, strangers.
2–3 years → fear of the dark, animals, thunder
5–8 years → fear of monsters, TV creatures, ghosts
9–12 years → fear of injuries, disasters
Adolescents → fear of failure, criticism (social evaluative fears)

75. C. Child who obeys the rules laid by teachers has reached the preconventional stage 1 of Jean Piaget's theory

Option A refers to the latency stage of Freud's psychosexual stages. This stage is 5/6 to 11/13 years. It corresponds to the industry versus inferiority stage of Erikson's theory of psychosocial development. In the preoperational stage, a child shows egocentrism, which refers to a child's restricted ability to view the world from another's point of view. This is evident from the mountain task. Fear of punishment and guilt is seen in the initiative versus guilt stage of Erikson, which corresponds to the phallic stage of Freud's psychosexual stages. In Mahler's differentiation stage, a child (5–10 months) starts differentiating mother from self; however, in the practising phase a child (10–18 months) gradually shows interest in the outer world and practises exploration.

76. B Some affection-deprived children are capable of forming attachments

Psychodynamic psychiatrists rely on historical data. The new work on effects of early life experiences postulate that few of these experiences are irreversible. Not all successful adults come from toxic homes but for some this may be the case. Many come from deprived or toxic homes and appear to be invulnerable to stresses. Freud postulated a universal sequence of emotional development (existence of infantile sexuality, attachment to primary caretaker, ubiquity of conflicts and jealousy in the family). However, the universal sequence did not find empirical support.

77. C Peer-only-reared primates are clingy and timid in their reactions to others

In total isolation the female is unable to nurture the young (motherless mother).

Mother-only reared fails to leave its mother and is terrified when exposed to its peers.

Choo-choo phenomenon: peer-only reared grasps others in a clingy manner, reluctant to explore, timid as an adult and play minimal.

In partial isolation self-mutilation and stereotyped behaviours are seen. There is initial protest, which changes to despair in 48 hours – seen in separation.

78. C Impersonality

When a crowd has gathered, LeBon (1879) noted that the behaviour is modified or influenced by several determinants in a particular situation. LeBon (1879) has described a high degree of suggestibility in a crowd as a result of which rumour becomes a significant part in influencing the behaviour. In addition, individuals in a crowd stimulate each other and work together in a 'social contagion'. If the situation is of riots and mobs, the crowd behaves in a manner where the members of 'enemy' are treated as equally bad. Furthermore, LeBon noticed that, when there is anonymity, the crowd assumes the role of moral responsibility, thereby shifting the sense of individuality from an individual to a crowd. In this situation, the action taken is greater than that by an individual.

79. E Two-sided presentations

In persuasive communication, there are key aspects relating to the message and attitude change, which include:

1. Message repetition can be a persuasive influence leading to attitude change.
2. Explicit messages are more persuasive for less intelligent recipients.

3. Implicit messages are more persuasive for more intelligent recipients.
4. Interactive personal discussions are more persuasive than mass media.
5. One-sided communications are more persuasive for those who are less intelligent and/or already favourably disposed to the message.
6. Two-sided presentations are more effective with intelligent and neutral recipients.
7. A low-anxiety recipient is more influenced by a high-fear message, and vice versa.

80. A Asch Experiment

The Asch conformity experiment showed the power of conformity in small groups.

Muzafer Sherif's robbers cave experiment worked on intergroup relationships. He divided people into two competing groups to explore how much aggression would emerge.

In Leon Festinger's cognitive dissonance experiment, people justified their lies by changing their previously unfavourable attitudes about the task.

The Milgram experiment studied how far people would go to obey an authority figure.

The bobo doll experiment by Albert Bandura has shown how aggressive behaviour is learned by exposure to media violence.

In the Stanford prison experiment, Philip Zimbardo demonstrated to what extent people would follow an adopted role.

81. B Precontemplation

According to Prochaska and DiClemente (1993), patients come to clinicians at different stages of readiness to make changes in their behaviours and habits. Motivation is not a fixed or unchanging entity, but it fluctuates from day to day and in different circumstances.

82. D Maintenance

According to Prochaska and DiClemente (1993), patients come to clinicians at different stages of readiness to make changes in their behaviours and habits. Motivation is not a fixed or unchanging entity, but it fluctuates from day to day and in different circumstances.

83. D Psychodynamic therapy

The focus of psychodynamic psychotherapy is understanding how past experiences influence present behaviours. It is a form of treatment that examines defence mechanisms, transference, and the internal world of fantasy and object relations. It also examines how unconscious mental functioning influences one's thoughts, feelings and behaviours. It can be subdivided into two sub-types: brief or time-limited therapy of up to 6 months or 24 sessions, and long-term or open-ended therapy.

84. D Middle session

The technique of psychodynamic psychotherapy has evolved from a largely silent and non-directive role for the therapist to one in which the therapist is lively and interactive. The interventions include observation, interpretation, confrontation, clarification, encouragement and empathic validation. Resistance means that the patient unconsciously resists psychotherapy because of ambivalence towards change. Defence mechanisms that have worked for many years are heightened when the psychic equilibrium is threatened by psychotherapy.

85. C Interpersonal therapy

This is a time-limited, diagnosis-based treatment developed by the late Gerald Klerman, and his wife Myrna Weissman and colleagues, for a clinical trial of the treatment of major depression. It is indicated for depressed adolescents, geriatric patients, depressed patients in primary care, depressed HIV-positive patients, depressed women in divorce disputes, pregnant and postpartum women, and non-depressed bulimic patients. Interpersonal therapy deals with grief, role disputes, role transitions and interpersonal deficits.

86. B Primary prevention aims at reducing the prevalence of hazardous drinking or the hazards of drinking

Primary prevention can be achieved by three strategies: control of availability, education about sensible use and providing alternative pursuits. Secondary prevention aims to prevent further progression of a condition by identifying and treating cases at an early stage. It can be achieved by harm minimisation.

87. D Kraepelin

The term 'dementia precox' was coined by Kraepelin. Bleuler coined the term 'schizophrenia'.

Hecker coined the term 'hebephrenic schizophrenia'. Morel coined the term 'dementia précoce'. Kahlbaum coined the term 'catatonia'. Kraepelin distinguished between manic depression and dementia precox, which was later named schizophrenia.

88. E Morel

Benedict Morel (1809–1873) was a French psychiatrist; he used the term 'dementia précoce' to describe the group of patients who had deteriorating mental illness that started in adolescence.

89. C 1933

In 1933, Jacob Kasanin introduced the term schizoaffective disorder to refer to the condition, which has symptoms of both schizophrenia and affective disorder. From 1933–1970, the patients who had similar symptoms of Kasanin's patients were classified as schizoaffective disorder.

90. B Displacement

This involves the resolution of the conflict about some particular relationship or event by shifting emotion attached to it onto some other relationship or event that is perceived as less threatened.

91. D Repression

This involves suppressing from awareness emotions and memories experienced as painful. It happens to protect the psyche, and overlaps with denial.

92. B Altruism

Altruism is a type of higher or mature defence mechanism. In this, a person deals with inner conflict or any stress by helping others or fulfilling the needs of others. Sublimation is the transformation of the instinctual energy to a more socially acceptable one. Reaction formation is seen in the patients with obsessive–compulsive disorder; here the attitude is opposed to the oppressed wish and constitutes the opposite reaction. Humour is also a mature defence in which a person deals with stress by giving it a humorous form or takes things lightly in a jovial way.

93. B Projection

Projection: unacceptable thoughts, emotions and feelings are projected on some other person.

Repression is a type of basic defence in which unacceptable or uncomfortable Ideas, thoughts or emotions are pushed away into the unconsciousness.

Rationalisation is a way of explaining the things more logically, and in a socially acceptable way so that the true motive is not perceived. For example, a heavy drinker explains the cardiac advantage of drinking alcohol.

94. D Personality disorder

In the DSM-IV, schizotypal disorder is part of personality disorders whereas in the ICD-10 it is part of schizophrenia spectrum disorders.

The DSM-IV categorisation of schizotypal disorder as a personality disorder is controversial.

95. E Selective abstraction

Selective abstraction is focusing on one aspect of an event and ignoring the more important features, as in the case of this footballer, who is ignoring all his capabilities and focusing on one failure.

Concentrating on the worst-case scenario or outcome of a situation is catastrophic thinking. Black-and-white thinking is also called dichotomous thinking, in which a person thinks all or none. Rationalisation and projection are defence mechanisms and not the cognitive distortions or biases.

96. E Kasanin

The term 'schizoaffective psychosis' was coined by Kasanin. In 1933, Jacob Kasanin introduced the term 'schizoaffective disorder' to refer to the condition that has symptoms of both schizophrenia and affective disorder. From 1933 to 1970, the patients who had similar symptoms to Kasanin's patients were classified as schizoaffective disorder.

97. C Jules Falret

In 1984, Jules Falret described the condition associated with alternating moods of depression and mania. He called it folie circulaire. It was Hippocrates who used the terms such as 'mania' and 'melancholia' to describe mental illness. Kahlbaum used the term 'cyclothymia'. Kraepelin coined the term 'dementia precox'.

98. C They extend beyond young adulthood

Erikson's stages do embrace some concepts of infantile sexuality and give importance to events outside oneself. However, it differs from Freud's ideas because it proposes developmental stages up to old age.

99. A Classification of neurology

Although Charcot is associated with hypnosis, he is best known for his work classifying neurological signs and symptoms, and making neurology a modern scientific discipline.

Luigi Galvani demonstrated nerve–muscle conduction.

No one person is credited with discovering neurotransmitters.

The Austrian physician Anton Mesmer was the first to practise hypnotism on patients with hysteria.

100. D Preoperational stage

Semiotic function or the ability to represent objects with a signifier appears in the preoperational period.

101. A An absence of adolescent turmoil such as competitiveness/aggression

Margaret Mead described how the Samoan society condemned aggressiveness and nurtured relationships, encouraging communal rearing of children. This helped to cement the beliefs of cultural determinism as opposed to biological determinism. But her findings were later proved false and her methodology flawed.

102. B Characteristics of human communication systems

Karl Von Frish studied communication in bees which prompted studies of human communication.

Aggression: Konrad Lorenz studied aggression in animals

Attachment/social deprivation: studied by Harlow using monkeys

Stress: Pavlov also studied stress and neurosis in animals along with Gantt and Liddell in the USA.

103. E Statute law

This is made via a legislative process carried out by parliament. Common or case law applies to similar cases that have been processed legally in the past and is also known. Criminal law deals with offences that are deemed punishable by common law, statute law or a regulation from a subordinate authority. Civil law is related to non-criminal activity.

104. D Negative autoscopic hallucination

Negative autoscopy is a phenomenon wherein the person is unable to see his or her own reflection in the mirror.

- Hypnagogic hallucination: hallucinations occurring just before sleeping.
- Hypnopompic hallucination: vivid dream-like hallucination that occurs as one is waking up.
- Hygric hallucination: hallucination of water or fluid perceived in a tactile modality.

105. B Decreased slow wave sleep

In depression, there is evidence to suggest that there is decreased slow-wave sleep, decreased delta waves and increased total REM sleep. There is decreased latency to REM sleep.

106. C The infant splits his or her experiences into 'good' and 'bad' elements of the mother and him- or herself

Children realise that their mother has both positive and negative aspects: depressive position.

An infant projects feelings of rage and hatred on to the mother and fears the same feelings from the mother: projective identification.

The infants fear attack from the 'bad' mother – persecutory anxiety.

Unconscious knowledge of bodily functions – phantasy.

107. B Carl Rogers

- Major concepts of person-centred theory are self-actualisation and self-direction.
- Adolf Meyer introduced the idea of common-sense psychiatry.
- Harry Stack Sullivan introduced modes of experiencing the world – proto taxic mode, parataxic mode and syntaxic mode.
- Sartre: introduced existential psychoanalysis.
- Otto's rank introduced birth trauma as the origin of anxiety.

108. E Sodium valproate

This has a high absorption of moisture when exposed to moist air or humidity. Hence, it must be stored in airtight containers or its original packaging. It is a white, odourless, crystalline powder with a saline taste. It is highly soluble in water and alcohol.

109. C Jung described the concept of the collective unconscious

This includes archetypes. Jung did not agree with Freud's theories of infant sexuality. He described the anima and animus, which are the undeveloped feminine and masculine qualities in men and women respectively. Jung was very much influenced by eastern mysticism and the therapeutic goal was to achieve individuation.

110. B Hippocrates

In 1984, Jules Falret described the condition associated with alternating moods of depression and mania. He called it folie circulaire. It was Hippocrates who used the terms such as 'mania' and 'melancholia' to describe mental illness. Kahlbaum used the term 'cyclothymia'. Kraepelin coined the term 'dementia precox'.

111. C Brown and Harris

In 1978, Brown and Harris published their influential book on the social origins of depression. They argued that depression was primarily caused by psychosocial factors. They suggested that events with severe and long-term, threatening implications that involved loss played a major role in the aetiology of depression. They pointed towards the class differences in the prevalence of depression, with working class women five times more likely to develop depression after a major life event.

112. B Intoxication occurs soon after consumption of alcohol

Intoxication occurring soon after consumption of alcohol is part of pathological intoxication. The other symptoms forming some of the criteria for alcohol intoxication are disinhibition, aggression, impaired attention and judgement, and difficulty in standing.

For alcohol intoxication, there ought to be at least one dysfunctional behaviour and one sign among the three, i.e. unsteady gait, slurred speech and difficulty in standing.

113. C Concomitant use of serotonin selective reuptake inhibitors can lead to the serotonin syndrome

Abrupt withdrawal of lithium has been associated with a rapid onset of mania, although, generally, there is an increased risk of recurrence of mood disorder on stopping lithium.

Concomitant use of angiotensin-converting enzyme (ACE) inhibitors results in increased lithium levels, and hence the risk of toxicity. Other drugs that increase lithium levels are non-steroidal anti-inflammatory drugs (NSAIDs) and antibiotics such as metronidazole. Diuretics lead to an increase in lithium levels. Furosemide is, by far, the safest diuretic with lithium.

Drugs such as theophylline and sodium bicarbonate reduce lithium levels.

Concomitant use of serotonin selective reuptake inhibitors can lead to the serotonin syndrome.

114. E Thomas Szasz

Thomas Szasz said 'Is there such a thing as mental illnesses?'

RD Laing and Michael Foucault are known for the anti-psychiatry movement.

L Ron Hubbard started the scientology movement.

David Cooper coined the term 'anti-psychiatry'.

115. C European court

According to the doctrine of precedence a decision by a higher court according to a hierarchy is binding over the decision of a lower court. The hierarchy from least to most binding is shown in **Table 5.4**.

Table 5.4 Courts in the UK and Europe in ascending order of higher court
1. Magistrates court
2. Crown court
3. High court
4. Court of appeal
5. Supreme court
6. European courts

116. C 3.6 times

David et al (1995) investigated the association of left-handedness, epilepsy and hearing impairment with schizophrenia in the cohort study of 50,000 male Swedish conscripts, linked to the Swedish National Register of Psychiatric Care. The study revealed that schizophrenia was higher among those with severe hearing loss.